The Complete
LOW CARB
HIGH FAT
NO HUNGER DIET

A User Manual for Our KetoHybrid Diet
Constructed from the Best Practices of
Low Carb, Ketogenic, & Paleo-Inspired Diets

by Veronica Childs and Laura Childs

Hula Books
Delhi ~ Canada

Canada – USA – UK – India – Ireland
New Zealand - Australia – South Africa

editor@hulabooks.com
www.hulaboks.com

Published by Hula Books (Canada)
Suite #872, 693 Peel Street
Delhi N4B2H3

Printed in The United States of America

Book Design by Laura Childs
Editing and Recipe Creation by Veronica Childs
Dessert Recipe Consultations with Madison Zelkowicz

ISBN-10: 1499793251
ISBN-13: 978-1499793253

We dedicate this book to
every woman and man
who questions the
standards and
seeks the
truth.

Table of Contents

Entrees & Dinner Ideas--139

Vegetable Entrees and Side Dishes------------------------------163

Acknowledgments

We would like to thank all of our friends for their continued encouragement throughout this process. We hope that we have inspired you as much as you have inspired us!

We both would like to thank a wonderful father and even better husband – Eric Kleinoder. He put up with our tears and rants over weight gain, celebrated in our triumphs, and ate all of the test kitchen's concoctions; both good and bad.

A special thank you must be noted to Madison Zelkowicz for lending a hand in the test kitchen. Without this trained pastry chef modifying our recipes we might have been sharing cardboard creations. To sample Madison's best, you have to try the Mini Chocolate Cheesecake just once.

We are also extremely grateful for Tim Castleman (Texas) for his business and marketing advice and coaching. Without Tim's guidance we might have been years in releasing this information.

We are also happy to acknowledge the many authors and scientists that contributed to our research and understanding of human nutrition. How could we thank them all? Over time, we will review each book and research study on our website in an effort to gain more exposure for each of them. Our aim will be that this research, ideals and news, reach many others in their quest for weight loss and optimum health.

Most of all, we would like to thank and acknowledge you. You are making our dream possible – to reach and assist as many people as we can. Please share this book with your friends. Please share your weight loss success story with us. Your own story could inspire hundreds, even thousands of others who are suffering because of a few extra pounds. We will be setting up a space on the website for you. In the meantime, our email is always open to accept your note.

INTRODUCTION

Welcome in the new, thinner, you! Do it right now because this diet's typical results will have you seeing losses on that bathroom scale in as little as three days.

Three days to first results is the reason we could wait no longer to share this with you. We are certain that once you see results, continuing on and eventually making this a lifestyle choice becomes an easy decision to make.

This diet is neither challenging nor complicated. If you're in a rush to get started you'll find our helpful 10-step quick start and choose to learn more as you find the time.

Your early results won't just show up on the scale. Yes, you will lose weight without hunger, but you'll also notice results in inches lost. By the tenth day, you should also note an increase in energy.

With all the benefits to this diet, you may wonder why no one else is talking about this and why you hadn't started sooner. Perhaps you didn't know that losing weight could be so easy, could be achieved without hunger, or that food allowed on a weight loss diet could taste this good.

This isn't your fault.

Until just recently only a small group of people have worked with a low carb high fat diet and even fewer are sharing their results.

You also need to know that some of the extra pounds you carry are also not your fault.

We - meaning millions of us - have been lied to. We have been told that foodstuffs in our stores and shelves are safe to eat. It's not. Many products and ingredients are responsible for weight gain and this information has been kept from the general public.

These trade secrets, fillers in foodstuff, effect on our bodies, go far beyond the total calories and serving sizes of packages.

Still, we're told by the diet gurus and our doctors to count our calories.

Told to banish all fat from our diets.

Told to starve ourselves skinny.

Essentially, to never enjoy a meal again.

When you follow their silly rules and lose the weight, it isn't long in returning. You know it's true, you've been there. So have we.

As for the weight returning – again, not entirely your fault.

We are fed such a massive heap of misinformation and at such a frenzied pitch, that we have no choice but to buy into it all.

Here's an example:

> *Your fit best friend, a television doctor, and the latest diet book all state that egg yolks contain fat and shouldn't be eaten. What do we do? We toss the yolks like they're poison.*
>
> *Two years later – growing frustrated with boring omelets, tasteless sauces, minimal weight loss, and half of your grocery dollars washed down the drain – the doctors, and the books, and the fit friend, apologetically change their tune.*
>
> *"Whole eggs are complete protein," they wail, "whites and yolks should be eaten together," and finally, "your body needs the fat of the yolk."*

No wonder so few diets have sustainable results or a following of folks still enjoying their meals!

Listen, you've been lied to about the safety of foods on the shelf. You've been lied to about percentages and suggestions for healthy daily intake. And you've only ever been given parts of the weight loss puzzle. This is especially true if you, like us, have been on a roller coaster ride with your weight.

Please understand that I am not suggesting that diets are purposefully misleading, or that they don't work, or are incorrect in their approach. Each one contains a part of the puzzle that makes the diet work. Each one offers you a deeper understanding of how your body works.

The trouble is that you have to sift through a mountain of books and research to discover which parts of the puzzle are doing all the work!

Imagine if a puzzle piece from each of the most successful diets worked nicely together.

Imagine that these pieces could create one easy plan making weight loss practically effortless, with quick results, and that the approach was conducive to the average person's life. A person who, like us, has minimal time to fuss with calories and restrictions and shopping for hard to find items. A person who still wants to take part in one of life's greatest joys – food!

That is what we imagined and how we came to realize that only a hybrid (parts of multiple) diet could solve our weight problem in a manageable and sustainable way.

We assessed multiple diets – why they worked and if they would work over the long term. We read countless research studies on the human body and weight loss.

We started poking around in common food additives business. We thought about the number of hours most people had available to look after their health and nutrition. Finally, we pieced the whole mess together into one cohesive diet, and we followed it through.

Our results speaks volumes for our methods.

We want those results, or better, for you!

We're making a commitment to share every secret, every piece of the puzzle, and bare our own souls to get you to your goal weight!

We're going to fill up the pages of this book with as much information as we can in the shortest amount of time.

As soon as this book is published we will begin supplementing even more nutritional information and weight loss research on our website. We want you to always have a resource you can trust.

We invite you to our conversation. We count you as part of our family. We hope that you will tell us if there's something here you just can't make sense of; if you do, we will look for an alternate way to explain it.

For lack of a catchier name, we've called this the **KetoHybrid Diet**.

What you need to know before you get started is that every aspect of this diet is grounded in science, has been backed by research, and has measurable results.

Each component has validity – yet those components have never been put together in this way. It is the balance of those components that will drive your results. We invite you to find that balance, lose the weight you want to lose, by learning about the KetoHybrid Diet. We hope you'll become our next success story!

We want you to know that even if you've tried dieting in the past, this diet is different.

The food is delicious and need never be boring. This is a way of eating that will train your body to burn excess fat with foods that will provide more energy and mental clarity than you've perhaps had in years.

Truly, the most important change of all isn't far from your reach; the emotional and mental shift that comes with each success. That sense of accomplishment; the increase in confidence when the scale takes that first dip or when the first outfit from your closet effortlessly slides over your body. When you are no longer nagged by the "feed me" voice; or when you head out for a shopping spree because your pants are falling off at work. (That actually happened!)

All we ask is that you trust us. That you move boldly through the first two weeks. As you do, you will change – on the outside as well as on the inside.

We can hardly wait to welcome the new, thinner, you!

Who We Are

We are you.

Unless you have a major health concern, there will be very little you can say to convince us that your challenges are any different than ours were at the start of this diet.

We are a mother and daughter, aged 50 and 20 respectively. We have been both fit and obese throughout the years. We are both stressed by bills, and car repairs, and every other worry of modern life.

Our head shots are below. Weight and bloat and unhappiness show on our 'before' faces. We will be posting full body before and after shots on the website shortly. There aren't many of Laura at her largest when she wasn't hiding behind a Christmas tree. Veronica was notorious at her largest for grabbing people's phones and immediately deleting any photos of her.

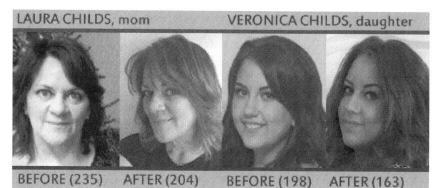

LAURA CHILDS, mom   VERONICA CHILDS, daughter

BEFORE (235)   AFTER (204)   BEFORE (198)   AFTER (163)

Laura (50, mother) works at her computer desk all day, and often through most evenings. She is, by choice, an insomniac. At her last doctor's visit (the 50 year marker), she was informed that she was only a few pounds away from being morbidly obese. She was warned that she displayed the early signs of metabolic syndrome (pre-diabetes). Laura is 5' 11" tall.

Veronica (20, daughter) works as a Manager in a retail store. She devotes 45-55 hours per week to the job and is on call during all business hours. She carries the worries of her store, her staff, daily sales, and the world at large on her shoulders – always has. Leaving home for college at 17 years old, she gained the traditional "Freshman 30". She continued to gain weight after entering the work force full time.

At the time of starting this diet Veronica was commuting over three hours per work day. Until just recently, Veronica wasn't even able to even a leg into her high school jeans. Veronica is 5' 7" tall.

As you can see, we are very different from each other, but we both had lifestyle challenges and were in agony over our size.

We have tried diets, exercise routines and lifestyle changes. Each change began with hope but brought a new misery.

We felt deprived, bordered on depression, and we were hungry.

We didn't have 1-3 hours per day to allocate to working out.

At times we would see a slight loss on the scale – but it was never worthy of our efforts and certainly never sustainable for the long term.

In frustration we would return to our old habits and gain the weight back.

More weight, every time.

As we write this we are saving up our dollars for professional full body 'after' photos and will be posting them on the website. In the meantime, you'll find some unprofessional ones taken with our cell phones.

You can connect with us at any of the links below or use the contact form on our websites.

http://www.lowcarbhighfatdiets.com
http://www.ketohybrid.com
https://www.amazon.com/dp/B00KNE08XW
http://www.facebook.com/lowcarbhighfatdiets
http://www.google.com/+Lowcarbhighfatdiets1
http://www.instagram.com/lowcarbhighfatdiet
http://www.pinterest.com/lowcarbdiets

Now let's get you started on our KetoHybrid diet.

HOW TO GET
A 2 WEEK MEAL PLAN... FREE
OR 20 MORE RECIPES...

Send a photo of yourself holding this book and we'll send along your choice of either book for free!

Get The Details - www.KetoHybrid.com/freebook

CHAPTER 1

What You Can Expect From KetoHybrid

Assuming you're relatively healthy, have visited your family doctor in the past 6 months, are between the ages of 20 and 50, have 15-80 pounds to lose (without jeopardizing your health), and you're not on life-saving medications, let's cover what you can expect and what is required to succeed with KetoHybrid.

First and foremost, you need to approach this diet with a little determination. For the majority, that dogged determination will only be required for the first three days. From that point onwards, your steady progress will fuel your journey.

The First Three Days

What's so hard about the first three days?

Breaking habits. Learning new ways to cook or order food. Overcoming an addiction to carbohydrates.

What's the worst that can happen in the first three days?

Potentially, a little fatigue and some cravings. A dull headache. Irritability. A slight decrease in mental alertness. It all passes.

What if I don't make it to the third day?

Then you pull up your socks and start again. You don't give up on the diet. You certainly don't give up on yourself. If it takes you seven days to get past day three, then so be it, but you keep trying. If you get to ten days and you don't think you'll ever make it past the first marker then you email either one of us and we'll give you some tips. Seriously though, you can do this. Put those three days behind you as quickly and as efficiently as you can.

What do I have to do?

Consciously cut carbohydrate intake to thirty net grams per day and drink enough water to start flushing out the toxins of our modern diets.

During this time you'll be breaking a cycle of addiction – addiction to sugar, to empty carbs, and to chemical additives. We'll talk about water intake and net grams of carbohydrates in the next chapter – neither requests are unreasonable.

The Remainder of the First Two Weeks

With the first three days under your belt (and I'll bet a few pounds flushed away), the worst is over.

The rest of this diet won't be as hard as those first few days, so give us another eleven days.

By two weeks in you can expect results, you will have gained the knowledge on why KetoHybrid works, and you feel enough new-found confidence that you won't be returning to your old diet.

At the two week mark, KetoHybrid becomes a lifestyle choice. It was at this point that we both said "Why would I ever want to do, or eat, any other way?"

Without getting ahead of ourselves, here's what you can expect.

Results: Substantial loss of pounds and some inches, without hunger, without excessive fussing in the kitchen, or keeping a food journal. An average weight loss of 8-15 pounds is expected, half of which may be loss of water retention, but don't discredit it. That water loss is the first step and a direct result of stored fat shrinking in size.

At Weeks Three & Four

A substantial decrease of inches – usually from the fattiest part of the body but varies per individual. Continued moderate weight loss with a minimum expectation of 3 pounds per week. Maximum is dependant on how much weight you have to lose and your adherence to the recommendations.

How You'll Feel: No hunger. An increase in energy. Improvement in sleep habits. A more positive mental state stemming from personal empowerment by gaining control over weight and the 'food loop'.

At Weeks 5 and Beyond

Continued effortless weight loss of 3+ pounds per week as well as inches over all body parts. Excess carb consumption is no longer considered a pleasurable experience, treat, or reward. An over-indulgence could make you feel ill. How do I know? I'm a cheater!

The Weight Loss Plateau

A perfect dieter, following the rules of a perfect diet – will still hit a plateau. Women suffer plateaus more often then men due to monthly hormonal changes as well as age-related hormonal changes.

Women are also more affected emotionally by a plateau – which just stalls us further.

There are many possible reasons for a plateau. Not all can be immediately rectified. Sometimes you just have to stay the course, wait it out, and don't let it stress you out. Stress hormones signal your body to hold onto fat reserves. Worrying about a plateau is the absolute worst thing you could do.

We both hit a stall at week #5. Mom started losing again after a three consecutive day increase in exercise (one hour moderate-paced walk each day). Veronica increased water intake for three days (20 ounces extra each day) to break the plateau.

If you'd rather be pro-active about a plateau and you like to experiment, here are some common hacks to get your body back into fat burning mode. None of these will cause you harm – even the suggestion of increasing your fat macro. Less familiar terms are explained in later chapters.

- Decrease portion size/overall calories by 20%.
- Increase water intake by 20%.
- Adding in light exercise.
- Assess daily intake (look for carb creep and/or balance macros).
- Increase fat percentage by 5% for a few days.
- Give intermittent fasting a trial run.

Cheating and Personal Fortitude

Cheat days or cheat meals within diets are common. These exist to ease a dieter's angst, to provide freedom during special events, and sometimes to snap the metabolism into high gear.

We understand that getting settled into a new diet might take a month. During that time cheating might even be accidental. Still, we can't suggest it as good dietary practice.

Did we cheat?

Heck yes we did! Did it break a plateau, or make us feel better, or speed up weight gain the following week? No. No it didn't. Our tests (for lack of a better word) resulted in two setbacks. First, we stalled our loss for a few days. Secondly, we noticed the return of cravings.

Should you cheat?

You will need to weigh the pros and cons and decide what is best for you. If the deal breaker for staying on the diet is going to be over a bag of pretzels, then eat the darn things. Just know that you might be kicking yourself for a few days after.

If you can hold out until you've met your target weight, then please do. You'll get to your target goal quicker and you'll gain new confidence based on the depth of your resolve.

Can you ever eat that bag of pretzels?

We believe you can. In moderation. On occasion. Once you have met your goal.

Since KetoHybrid alters the way your body burns food for energy, it is, in a real sense, a metabolic reset. Also, once you are comfortable with the knowledge of how your body uses food, you'll know the best time to indulge in pretzels, or cake, or whatever your favorite cheat is.

For even more inspiration, understand that the majority of dieters who chose to remain on a plan long after they've met their goal weight are not as strict about their intake as they were in the beginning. You'll be able to cut yourself a lot more slack in the future.

In the grand scheme of life; setting yourself back a few days when you've already made great progress and know that you will continue on in your diet, isn't that big of a deal. If it takes you eight weeks instead of four to settle into this lifestyle, that's okay.

As your understanding of nutrition is altered, so will your relationship with food. It is an ongoing process until the day we die.

Success in anything is not measured by how quickly you can make a change, but by your continual progress, the increase in awareness, and by your fortitude.

Common Knowledge On Modern Foods

To ensure we're on the same page, let's quickly cover some common knowledge about modern food and nutrition.

If any concepts in this section are new to you, please take a few minutes at the end of this section to either research them or send us a note for clarification. We trust that these things are widely understood and don't want to waste your time going over each item. It is important however, that you believe these things to be true.

- Snacking after dinner is bad.
- A fast food lifestyle will lead to obesity, illness and potentially an early death.
- Factory-made foods are not really food at all. They are laboratory experiments that – when eaten by humans or lab rats – turn into overhangs and unhealthy organs.
- Some of the simplest and traditionally healthy foods in the grocery store are no longer healthy for human consumption.

- Fruits, vegetables, dairy products, fish, meats and more have now been altered or are being farmed in ways that make us gain weight, get sick, die young, or three.
- Farmed foods are over-sprayed with pesticides, genetically modified, bleached, over-processed, injected with hormones and antibiotics and treated to remain fresher, longer on the shelves. And all of that modification and 'extra' treatment is considered safe by our governments.

You knew all that right? You knew it and kept eating it even though the long term side effects are known to be devastating. You, like us, have been eating this way because you either didn't know you had a reasonable choice or that it really was all that bad for you.

You do have a choice. And yes, those foods and their 'extras' are that bad for you.

A few years ago the views above were considered 'fringe'. Organic farmers and their customers were considered extremists. Sometimes even scoffed at for not being with the times.

Today these views (and the horrifying results of our modern progress) are mainstream. The havoc we've created on our food supply is well known. It shows up in the evening news, in the tabloids, on reality TV shows, and is shared as distressing images on every social network online.

Up until this moment you may have felt powerless to make a change. Sure we can all sign a few online petitions. We can make vow to never buy that brand of chicken again. But at the end of the day, we're still hungry!

We're always hungry. Unnaturally hungry, in fact. We're hungry because our diets no longer contain life-sustaining food. We're hungry because even our 'good' food doesn't have the nutrient value it did just a generation ago.

Most of all, we're hungry because even though the modern diet has changed, our basic genetic profile has not.

Do you really want to know how this diet is going to change your eating habits? You're going to look at food in a whole new light. It won't be your comfort, it will be your sustenance. Your body is going to be a temple and you're only going to give it the best that you can afford.

Eating will no longer be about satisfying only your tongue, but about feeding muscle, and repairing cells, and helping your heart stay young. The end result of this diet is a love and respect for your body – there's no escaping it.

Real Life Examples, A 20 Year Old & A 50 Year Old

We neglected to measure ourselves before we started on KetoHybrid. Honestly, we didn't imagine it would work this well or that we'd one day want to write a book about it!

The measurements below start on Week 4 and show up to Week 13. Veronica started following the diet protocols on January 15th. Laura didn't start until February 4th but measured at the same time and marked as the same weeks as Veronica's. When we began we were weighing ourselves on two separate scales – Veronica's at her house, Laura's at her own. Partway through we switched to weighing in on a new and better quality scale.

We apologize if the way we measured is confusing but we need to be perfectly honest with you on our documentation and proof – it wasn't very organized! These aren't clinical trials after all; simply our very messy notes and record keeping.

At the end of the day we've realized that our numbers have never defined us. The way we feel about our size, the way our clothes fit now, and the increased confidence in knowing we can manage our weight by eating the right foods, are worth more to us!

At the time of publishing this book, we continue to eat the KetoHybrid way. Neither one of us are in any rush to lose the final pounds to our goal weight because we know the rest will come and we currently feel great. With that said Veronica has plans to lose another 8-10 pounds over the next 4-6 weeks; Laura wants to lose another 15-19 pounds over the next two months.

Please understand that we have not yet bothered ourselves about portion control or counting calories, even though we will discuss these. We also cheat from time to time, sometimes accidentally.

We are both embarrassed to share these numbers publicly, so I do hope they inspire you!

	Bust	Waist	Hips	Pounds	Week/Date
Veronica 20 years old				198	START Jan 15
	40	32	42	181	#4 Feb 10
	39	33	41	180	#5 Feb 19
	38	32	40	179	#7 Mar 4
	37	29	37	170	#9 Mar 19
	37	28	36	168	#10 Mar 28
	35	25	33	163	#13 Apr 18
Laura 50 years old				235	**START** Feb 4
	46	42	48	222	#4 Mar 4
	45	40	46	220	#6 Mar 19
	44	39	45	215	#7 Mar 28
	42	38	43	210	#10 Apr 18
	39	37	40	204	#13 May 10

CHAPTER 2

KetoHybrid Basics

In this diet we take the best of the top three diets – Ketogenic, Low Carb and a Paleo-inspired diet – and merge them together to create one easy to love, fat-burning diet.

Usually, your body converts the foods you eat: sugars, starches, carbohydrates, and even some of the protein and fat, into glucose (sugar). It then uses the glucose for energy. All your processes – thinking, moving, breathing, hormonal, metabolic, and more – use this glucose energy source. Unused glucose is stored away for later use in the form of fat cells.

Your body can also burn lipids (fat) for energy. All your bodily processes – all of them – can be run on lipids. This is not a new concept to science, the medical industry, or your body. We do not need to trick the body to burn fat for energy. We merely have to remind it to do so, force it to do so, by no longer feeding it foods that are easily converted into glucose. This is a re-training of sorts. Burning fat instead of glucose is as old as a caveman's feast-or-famine life cycle, built directly into our instincts and DNA.

I know, I said the F-word. Famine. Just a few pages after promising you that you'd never be hungry...

The truth is, you won't be hungry, but your body will attempt to notify you through cravings that it is missing a major component of its standard diet.

To re-train your body to burn lipids instead of glucose we starve it of carbohydrates. This forces the body to look elsewhere for energy. Since the human body is lazy, it takes the next easiest process - burning up existing muscle tissue. This is why so many dieters lose muscle tone by the end of other diets. We combat this problem before it starts by balancing your food intake. A properly balanced diet won't allow excessive loss of muscle. You will be maintaining most of your muscle tone and structure, while losing fat.

Therein lies the first glorious difference between a low fat diet and a high fat one.

A low fat, low calorie diet starves the body of fats and proteins and is largely comprised of carbohydrates. The body continues to operate on carbohydrates but burns through muscle to get the energy it requires.

A Low Carb High Fat (LCHF) diet starves the body of easy energy, supports and feeds existing muscle by ensuring adequate amounts of protein, and provides enough fat to keep the entire body running smoothly.

KetoHybrid is a "low carb, high fat, adequate protein" diet that turns our bodies into fat burners!

Making KetoHybrid Work For You

While you may be in a rush to get this diet working for you, it is important that you understand the base concepts of KetoHybrid.

A Ketogenic diet is the backbone of this diet plan and is based on the completely normal process of ketosis (burning fat for energy). Once your body transitions to burning fat for energy – and if you aren't supplying enough fat through food – it begins to burn stored fat.

To get the body into ketosis, we minimize the supply of carbohydrates. This is the Low Carb aspect of KetoHybrid.

Finally, we take the concepts of whole, natural and organic foods from Paleo-inspired diets. These foods and food rules ensure that you sustain health while decreasing the damaging substances in modern foods that make our bodies gain or hold onto, excess weight.

When these three aspects are combined you will no longer be filling your body with harmful agents, you will be balancing blood sugar levels, you will burn and flush fats and toxins, and you may even be starving out the potential for cancer growth. (Some very promising research is in the works.)

We have provided a 10 Step Quick Start in a later chapter but we do urge you to at least skim each chapter, taking enough time to understand each concept thoroughly. This knowledge is provided to empower you, not to slow you down or fill up pages.

If you need help understanding any of the material, do not hesitate to email us for clarification. By doing so you will be influencing later revisions of this book and helping future readers.

Apart from the learning material in this book, knowing the net carb value of everything you eat is also important to your success. To help you become familiar with net carb values, we've included a list of some common foods in a later chapter.

You'll also find a chapter on sample meals, a meal plan, and a shopping list. We do not expect you to follow either of our samples. These samples worked for us because we fashioned them after our own tastes. We strongly encourage you to choose foods you love to eat and to cook for your own tastes. With that said, if you aren't used to cooking at home, can't imagine what types of food to eat, or if you just need a few ideas – we do hope it helps.

We want you to be concerned about balanced nutrition – namely vitamins and minerals required by your body. We do suggest a multi-vitamin and share a few generic supplements that we feel helped us in our transformations. We also urge you to pay close attention to your body (on this diet or any other). Vitamin and mineral deficiencies are almost always preceded by warning signs – some of which are listed for you in a later chapter.

The last section of this book contains our favorite recipes, some notes on the different food groups, and tips on cooking for your new fat-burning body.

Hybrid Reasoning: Top Three Diets

You may be wondering why we didn't just work through one single low carb, Paleo-influenced, or Ketogenic diet. These diets do have high success rates and each one is easy to understand - but were they sustainable? Or would they eventually lead to boredom and diet dissatisfaction?

Understand that for the purpose of brevity, I'm being uber-simplistic by the classifications and summaries below. These were our observations only and we are not attempting to discredit the concepts of any diet by sharing our opinion.

Paleo dieters seldom touch dairy and never touch meat that isn't organically raised. The online communities supporting the diet can be less than friendly to beginners with all the posturing and arguing over what is, and what is not Paleo. While the diet is restrictive and some of the communities less receptive to non-perfect Paleo, the diet offers some great principles when it comes to weight loss; even though weight loss is not the primary focus of the diet.

In low carb communities you will find a friendly, more supportive crowd, but you'll also find a lot of bad advice with no eye for the effect of additives in packaged goods. Many of these followers have been duped by foods labeled 'low carb'. Many companies that market to low carb dieters have been found to be less than truthful in their advertising and nutrition labeling. Low carb diets are primarily about restricting carbs with a secondary focus on caloric intake. This is a great concept with incredible results but by focusing on carb intake only, there isn't enough attention paid to balanced nutrition.

Of the three, the Ketogenic diet outperforms.

This diet has roots in ancient history but gained worldwide attention in the 1920s as a way to control epileptic seizures.

Knowledge of human metabolism and nutritional needs has made this diet easy to follow for treatments other than neurological disorders and obesity. Core concepts of the diet today remain similar to the original - simple and whole foods, albeit boring in its medical application.

We will be using various aspects from each of the three diet types. The fat burning Ketogenic Diet with supporting components of both low carb and Paleo-influenced diets.

At the base core of each, low carb and Keto could be classified as being low carb high fat; with Paleo being low carb, high protein. We fully expect Paleo extremists to argue with us on that one, but the originator of the Paleo Diet (Loren Cordain) clearly shows in the 2012 edition of his book, that Paleo is low carb, high protein.

Health Benefits Other Than Weight Loss

There's more to this diet than weight loss. After the first two weeks of changing your food source, processes other than fat-burning are going to be affected.

How about an increase in strength and agility? Many Ketogenic, *and* Paleo-inspired, *and* low carb dieters have naturally transitioned into body-building, marathon running, and weekend athletes. Since you'll be burning fat and not muscle, by the time you've met your goal weight you'll be primed to follow suit.

How about a clearer complexion? Stronger, healthier hair and nails? You won't realize the effects of dedication to this diet for at least three months, but trust me, it's coming. Laura noted a significant decrease in adult acne and firmer facial skin at the three month mark.

Your brain will function better too. The effect of blood sugar spikes takes a toll on mental processing. Kicking the carb habit alone facilitates an increase in clear and focused thinking. We also noted that past the first four weeks we became more consistently optimistic.

Aspects of this diet are also known to lower the risk of diabetes and defeat oncoming metabolic syndrome. Cutting out processed foods, additives, chemicals, and over-dosing on carbohydrates eliminates blood sugar spikes while increasing insulin resistance.

Your teeth will be happier as well. Less refined sugar means less tooth decay. It also lowers the risk or incidence of halitosis. Gum disease and tongue cancer are also reduced based on current research studies on the effects of diets high in refined sugar.

The biggest benefit – in my opinion – is that you will no longer feel hungry all the time.

Let's quickly look at some of the current research and medical conditions Ketogenic diets are associated with. It is important that you know how powerful and helpful this diet can be for more than just weight loss.

Current studies are examining the diet to address, correct, prevent, or treat:

- Amyotrophic Lateral Sclerosis (ALS),
- Autism,
- Alzheimer's,
- Cardiovascular Risks (to improve triglycerides, HDL and LDL cholesterol)
- Depression,
- Diabetes Mellitus (Type 2, Adult-Onset Diabetes, Insulin Resistance, Metabolic Syndrome, NIDDM, pre-Diabetes),
- Epilepsy,
- Head Trauma,
- Migraine Headaches,
- Neurological Disorders,
- Parkinson's Disease, and
- Polycystic Ovary Syndrome (PCOS).

A Ketogenic diet is also thought to be protective against strokes and more recently as a prevention or treatment for cancer. In a book on coconut oil we were introduced to the idea that cancer might be prevented through diet and weight management – and that cancer cells could potentially be starved out of a body.

Since current studies have already proven that cancer cells thrive on glucose; logic follows that any Keto diet (following the same glucose management principle) is at least preventative. See Thomas Seyfried's book "Cancer as a Metabolic Disease", and "The Ketogenic Diet: Uses in Epilepsy and Other Neurologic Illnesses"[1] and KetoHybrid[2] for updates on current research studies.

---

1   The Ketogenic Diet: Uses in Epilepsy and Other Neurologic Illnesses, http://www.ncbi.nlm.nih.gov/pmc/articles/PMC2898565/

2   www.KetoHybrid.com/cancer

Sobering, right?

I ask that you look again at the illnesses and diseases listed above. Not to praise a KetoHybrid diet, but to truly understand the severity of diseases that excess glucose causes to the human body.

The absolute brilliance here is that while you are:

- losing weight and feeling better on this diet,
- you will also be lessening your risk of obesity related illnesses,
- and you may be protecting yourself from future degenerative diseases,

...and you'll do it all without breaking a sweat!

CHAPTER 3

Balancing Carbs, Fat, & Protein

Once governments and professionals decided that the "calories in, calories out" theory was only part of the puzzle of weight management, and that the recommended Food Pyramid simply wasn't working for ample nutrition; we all began looking at food differently.

Today we use macro-nutrients to describe the energy-providing components of food. There are three macro-nutrients: fat, protein and carbohydrates. To maintain health, humans must eat essential fats and essential proteins. Carbohydrates on the other hand, are said to be unnecessary.

In their defense, carbohydrate-based foods carry essential vitamins and minerals that may not be found naturally elsewhere. They also convert quickly into glucose which our bodies use as energy. Our brains access and use that glucose to function but in the absence of carbs, our body can also create glucose by metabolizing protein and converting fats. It has now been proven that our brains can also function on ketones; the by-product of metabolizing fat (stored or consumed).

For North Americans, this should cause some pause.

If we have an obesity epidemic, and unused energy created from carbohydrates is turned to fat, and we don't need carbohydrates to sustain life, then:

> a) why is the USDA suggesting our diets be 66-78% carbohydrate-based, and

b) why is the new (2011) USDA nutrition model so similar (in macro-nutrient breakdown) to the 2005 version?

Conspiracy theorists surmise that carbs are an efficient way to keep tax-payers hungry for foods amply grown on our soil, while ensuring we don't live long enough to collect pension payments.

In fairness to the USDA, I have guesstimated macros based on their suggestions of nutrition. I'm neither the first nor the only one to do so. I'm also not the first to notice the discrepancies in nutritional calculation of recipes they post for constituents.

What Is A Macro (Do I Really Need To Know)?

Up until now we're been discussing macros as analysis to entire diets, but you'll also find them useful for assessing daily intake.
If you only have 10-20 pounds to lose, you may never need to assess or track macros in your personal plan, but you should be both aware of and comfortable with them.

Here are the macros of the healthiest diets (plus a few that could surely kill you off at a young age):

	% Protein	%Fat	%Carb
Hunter Gatherer Era	15	65	20
Average American Diet	20	30	50
Food Pyramid (USDA 2005)	20	12	68
Food Plate (USDA 2011)	22	14	64
Paleo Influenced Diets	35-40	40-45	15-20
Standard Ketogenic Diet	15-30	60-75	5-10
KetoHybrid Diet	15-20	60-70	5-15

The most popular low carb diet is based on carbohydrate tolerance and not macros.

Macros and Net Carbs in Real Life

Are you ready? This is where dieting goes from "ugh, a diet" to "OH, I get it! I can do this!"

First, let's be sure you know the difference between total carbohydrates and net carbohydrates. I didn't!

Total Carbs vs. Net Carbs

A carbohydrate may contain dietary fiber, sugar, or both. Since our body doesn't convert fiber into usable energy, we can subtract all fiber grams from a carbohydrate's total to arrive at the net carb value. This is also known as the 'functional carbohydrate' value.

As a singular example, whole grain wheat flour has 87 grams of carbohydrate per cup; 15 grams are fiber. Therefore whole grain wheat flour has 72 grams of net carbs per cup.

Most meat, poultry, and fish have zero carbs.

Many vegetables are under 4 net grams per cup.

Cream is low, but milk is high. The higher the fat % in cream, the lower the net carb count.

Ample Variety In 20 Net Carbs Daily

3 tbsp heavy cream (in coffee or tea)
2 eggs
3 slices of bacon
1/2 cup almond flour
1/2 cup raspberries
1 cup cauliflower
1 1/2 cups lettuce
1/2 cup green peppers
1/2 cup cherry tomatoes
4 oz Cheddar cheese
1 oz Macadamia nuts
1/2 avocado

Total Carbohydrates:	**39.29 grams**
Total Fiber:	**20.5 grams**
Total Net Carb:	**18.79 grams**

Many cheeses are quite low.

A list of net carb counts for common foods are shown in a later chapter. You'll also find carbohydrate breakdowns on nutrition labels, in books devoted to food counts, and through Google searches.

Sample Meals Based on Macros

Now let's examine how macros and net carbs convert to food equivalents in recipes and meals.

From this exercise you'll learn that you won't ever be hungry on KetoHybrid, you won't need to count calories as long as your macros measure up and you're eating to satiation, and that diet food needn't be boring.

To illustrate this, we only need to compare two meals from two diets – a USDA meal vs. a Paleo-inspired one.

Keeping in line with USDA's plating division plus ensuring adequate portion size, here's a spaghetti dinner built by macros.

> **Calories:** 360
> **Macros:** P: 28%; F: 11%, C: 61% (the closest I could get)
> **Net Carbs per Serving:** 49.0 grams
> 1 cup cooked whole wheat spaghetti
> 1/4 cup marinara sauce
> 1 oz ground chicken breast
> 1 oz mushrooms
> 1/6 ounce (light sprinkling) grated Parmesan cheese

Imagine that on your dinner plate!

Would you stop eating at one serving size? I probably wouldn't. I also know I'd be hungry again as soon as my body burned through all the carbs.

To be fair to the USDA, I took the time to test both the macros and calories for 5 random meals on their website[3].

A few that looked balanced, (and more palatable than the spaghetti dinner above), turned out to be quite different than their literature suggests. Fat macros as high as 33% go against what they preach. Their entrees – with net carbs in the 70 gram range and containing 14+ grams of sugar, yet considered to be only 28% of the recommended daily carb intake – are also disturbing.

---

3 www.myplate.gov

Bad advice aside, let's look at a Paleo-styled dinner plate.

> **Calories:** 367
> **Macros:** P: 40%; F: 43%; C: 17%
> **Net Carbs per Serving:** 10.9 grams
> 6 oz chicken breast
> 1 cup broccoli
> 1 cup Brussels sprouts
> Plus a salad that consists of:
> 2 cups lettuce
> 1/2 cup red pepper
> 2 tsp olive oil
> 1/4 tsp garlic

Although neither of these dinners might appeal to you, the points are clear regarding nutrition.

Neither healthful, interesting, nor satisfying nutrition is made by following USDA Guidelines. Most of us who have followed their guidelines (high carb, low fat) have ended up weighing more than we need to, eating more often than we should, and still feeling hungry for most of the day.

The Paleo-inspired meal above is reasonable, health sustaining, and sating. It feeds the body while restricting carbohydrates.

Understanding and Working With Macro-Nutrients

When we first started on the KetoHybrid journey, we didn't pay the slightest attention to our macro-nutrient levels.
We also didn't count calories, nor did we exercise portion-control.

We simply, drastically, cut carbs; made a concerted effort to eat more healthy fats more often; and didn't eat past the point of feeling full (this last point takes a while to master). The weight started coming off in record numbers for both of us.

Eventually, however, that party ends. When it does, you can't help but become interested in how to use food macros to move or keep yourself in ketosis – the state of which your body burns fat.

You already know that food contains macro-nutrients: fat, protein and carbohydrates.

And you know that food also contains important micro-nutrients: acids, minerals and vitamins.

You also have an ample knowledge regarding calories.

We're still going to talk about them all, just a little more.

While the caloric value of foods is important, that number isn't the star of the show.

That number won't tell you how the food will affect your body - knowing the macro breakdown would. This concept may be common knowledge, but it is often overlooked. Increasing your recommended daily intake with 500 calories of green beans won't have the same effect as doing so with a 500 calorie cupcake.

Unless you have hit a rock-solid plateau and haven't made a pound or an inch of progress for 10 days, don't fret the calories. You will make more progress and learn more about nutrition by giving your time and attention to the macros.

We "look after the macros and let the calories look after themselves."

When you look after the macros, a cupcake doesn't even cross your radar as food. The extra serving of green beans might though, and if you're hungry there is no hesitation or regret when adding it to your plate. (Green beans are just an example. When looking after the macros, you might be considering cheese, or an extra burger, or any other real food.)

Your Body On Macro-Nutrients

You'll see macros for food items displayed in the same manner as we used for the various diets on the previous page; P: #%, F: #%, C:#%.

It is the macro of a calorie – plus the way our body puts that macro-nutrient to use, plus our current engagement – that determines whether a calorie is detrimental or beneficial to our current health.

Theoretically, here is how our bodies uses the components of macro-nutrients:

- **Carb calories** are a good source of fiber and provide flavors and nutrients not found in other food types.
- **Excessive carb calories** (after being converted to glucose) will be stored as fat unless they are burned as energy (approximately 2 hours on either side of physical activity - engagement).

- **Protein calories** are used to build or repair muscle tissue. Protein can be converted to glucose which the brain may decide to put to use.
- **Excessive protein calories** converting to glucose can be stored as fat (plus other potential health complications).

- **Fat calories** carry fat-soluble vitamins (A, D, E and K) and minerals to your organs and cells. Fat feeds and supports all the processes in your body – from your metabolism to your fingernails. Fat calories leave you feeling fuller (sated), longer, as they are slow to digest.
- **Excessive fat calories** can also create bulk.

Therein lies most of the power of the KetoHybrid diet.

While every weight loss diet works by burning more calories than consumed, it is the macro-nutrient balancing of KetoHybrid that can easily keep you in a caloric deficit.

Balancing macros ensures minimal-to-zero carb-based calorie excess, while providing ample protein and fat calories.

No insulin spikes, no carbs creating new fat stores, no muscle loss, no insane hunger or uncontrollable cravings, and a metabolism that is passionate about running on fat (consumed or stored). All this, with a sated appetite!

You will, within a few days or a few weeks of eating a high fat diet, be eating less and thinking about food less often. In a month's time we may even need to remind you to eat. (It happened to us!)

Look After The Macros...

While we (and many others) don't track macros religiously, it is good practice.

Keeping tabs and knowing that you are on track will have immense value when you hit a plateau, when you are pondering a cheat food, or when you want to add more variety to your diet.

Tracking is easier than it sounds. It takes just 5 minutes of your day using the steps below.

You track all foods consumed over a 7-10 day period and then assess and adjust your diet based on what you learn. You might learn more about your eating habits, how your schedule affects your eating habits, discover where you've miscalculated certain foods, or find new ways within your diet to meet goals quicker.

What we don't want is to see you obsessing over perfect numbers. Strive for a range, not an absolute. Make feeding your body the first priority, optimum ranges the second.

"I don't want to track macros."

We didn't want to track macros either!

Veronica only considered her macros once and only because she had hit a plateau – she discovered that she was wasn't getting enough fat at that time and adjusted her intake. Laura checks macros more often. Lately she's found that while her carbohydrates are fine, her protein intake is low through the week (not so on weekends where meals are more traditional).

Can you see now how tracking macros is more conducive to personal tastes and daily habits than counting calories and feeling deprived?

Remember, one of the great features of following a KetoHybrid diet is that the secret sauce is in the balance. As long as you're losing weight or inches, you might never need to worry about watching those macros. On the other hand, if you don't know that you're balanced, you won't know if you're getting the best results.

You certainly can take our initial path (easy, but uncertain macro-balancing). This is your diet, your way. If you don't want to track macros right away, follow our 10 steps and don't worry about the macros until you need to – if you ever need to.

10 Step, Macro-Free, Quick Start

Here is how we started (plus a few tips we forgot early on):

1. Set a weekly weight loss goal for the first 4 weeks. We both wanted to lose at least 4 pounds per week even though we've been told that 2 pounds per week is optimal.

2. Weigh and measure yourself and write those numbers down in a place you won't lose them. Record the date as well as the time of day.

3. Prepare all your meals at home and bring your lunch to work. This saves you money, prevents needless temptations, ensures that you don't get hungry through the day, and minimizes the opportunities for legitimate mistakes. Don't buy or eat pre-made, fat-free, or low-fat foods.

4. Restrict your net carb intake daily until you're down to about 20 grams per day. This will take most of your focus in the first month. Carbs hide everywhere and in (nearly) everything!

5. Eat fat with every meal – fatty bacon, a tablespoon of coconut oil, mayonnaise, cheese, butter, olive oil, Hollandaise, etc. Put it on your food and don't worry that it will make you fat – it won't – it will feed you and start training your body to burn fat as an energy source.

6. Take a multi-vitamin with your meal; always with a fat source. A good vitamin – taken correctly – will help replace some of the vitamins and minerals you might be missing from carb restriction. Some essential vitamins are only fat-soluble (they won't be absorbed with a glass of water).

7. Drink 2-3 cups of home made broth (or at the very least bouillon) daily. Broth replaces electrolytes that might normally be found in carb-intake and adds more food to your daily diet without adverse effects.

8. Drink water or herbal teas throughout the day, all day.

9. Don't drink your carbs. Get the sugar out of your coffee. No fruit juices. No glasses of milk. Steer clear of sugar-free drinks (diet sodas, etc.) or any other sugar-free foodstuffs. (You may be able to add some sugar-free foods back in at a later date. You'll need to experiment and assess – but only once you're close to your goal.)

10. Assess your weight loss and measurements goals weekly. If you are on target – great! If you are not losing pounds and inches start tracking your macros and give a little attention to calories. And, since you're looking at your macros, take a moment to check over your micro-nutrients as well (to see if you need to add supplements to your diet).

The Five Minutes A Day Macro Track – Short Term

There are ample free smartphone apps and websites that help you track your daily food intake. Many are linked to the USDA nutritional database (values in the database are truer than the recipes they publish).

When you use these free services, your food entries will be automatically calculated for your three macro-nutrients (fat, protein, and carbs). These calculations will also show your calories and micro-nutrients – both worthy of contemplation.

Entering your daily food literally takes 5 minutes per day. It may take a little longer in the beginning and it will take longer if you are eating specialty gourmet dishes with multiple ingredients.

Be aware that most apps will be following the USDA's Food Guidelines (suggesting that you eat far more carbs and far less fat), and won't allow you to make custom changes to your macros. Don't worry about this and don't worry about their suggestions. You know the right macros to target. At a glance you'll know if you're in the right range.

	% Protein	%Fat	%Carb
KetoHybrid Diet	15-20	60-70	5-15

On Android devices and Windows-based computers, Laura uses MyFitnessPal. This service allows you to input your desired macros, track food intake, track weight loss, set up goals, and assess it all as often as you like. You do not need to share any of your information with the community, opt into any email updates, or track your physical activity if those features don't appeal to you.

On iOS (iPhone, iPad, and MacBook), Veronica has been using CalorieCount. This is a program that doesn't allow you to adjust your macros and tries to tell you where your diet is lacking. Veronica ignores their suggestions and keeps a watchful eye on macros and calories only. CalorieCount allows you to add your favorite foods, view your macros in a pie graph (by food item and by daily intake), and view calories consumed, quickly and easily.

Looking After & Adjusting Macros – Long Term

Looking after the macros becomes easier with time and practice; eventually becoming an on-going tabulation in your brain, the same as your bank account balance. If you don't consistently bounce checks, you likely won't need to track macros past the first 4-6 weeks.

At your goal weight, you have already established new eating habits. You know how your body feels at it's best. If you're still tracking macros daily by the gram, stop.

Too often, what innocently began as a 5 minutes per day awareness exercise, turns into an hour per day obsession. Don't let macro-balancing, calorie counting, and fractions of a pound stress you out or consume your life. You've met your goal, you know how to get back on track if you slip, so relax. Remember, stress steals your energy and makes your body hoard fat. Five minutes per day equates to over 30 hours at the end of the year. Half an hour a day is over 180 hours.

There is much more to learn about working with and balancing macros but unless you're working out at the gym or performing strenuous activities at work, you won't need to delve any deeper.

Unless, of course, you want to.

CHAPTER 4

Running on Fat – Understanding Ketosis

As stated earlier we are hard wired to burn fat for fuel. Our modern lifestyle, with ample supply of carbohydrate-based foods, seldom provides a reason for our bodies to put this talent into practice.

The state at which your body burns fat for fuel instead of glucose (from carbs) is called ketosis. Once in ketosis you are said to be fat-adapted, or even keto-adapted.

The transition takes an average of 7-10 days. It could be 3 days, it could be 3 months. To the best of my knowledge, no time-estimation criteria (age, BMI, sex, etc.) exists. You might experience negative symptoms until you are fully adapted. These seldom last past the initial seven days whether you are in ketosis or not.

If your diet was carb-heavy the first sign that you are in ketosis is the complete lack of cravings for empty carbs. Stay on track (no cheating) and you'll continue to burn fat for fuel. Some of us will be lucky – even a cheat day won't slip us out of ketosis.

During ketosis your liver will be breaking fat down into fatty acids and ketones – both of which will be used as energy. While most ketones head straight for the bloodstream, some will spill out through urine and saliva.

Here's where the processes of the human body can get a little tricky and where much misinformation exists. You already know that our bodies turn carbohydrates into glucose – to be used as energy. You also know that many experts state we don't need carbohydrates, even though we do need some glucose.

So where would that glucose come from if we didn't need or weren't eating enough carbs?

The Liver Converts Fat to Glucose

Our liver is capable of creating up to 150 grams of glucose per day from fat and protein. Sharing this information with others may spark a lively discussion. (I'm warning you in advance!)

While most nutritionists and medical doctors will agree that protein can be converted by the liver, the liver's ability to convert fat to glucose is not common knowledge – but it has been proven.

We are not attempting to discredit experts. Our desire is only to inform and set the record straight. Thousands of articles in journals and websites stating that our liver cannot convert fat are misleading and erroneous. The conversion is a lengthy and inefficient process (in comparison to the quick carb-to-glucose conversion), but extensive research has proven that it is so.

The most recent and extensive research shows 22 processes (pathways) exist to facilitate the conversion[4]. I apologize, but the research is beyond the scope of this book; as well as my ability to translate into conversational English. You will find others also sharing this new and valuable information – and doing a much better job of explaining it.

The Brain's Glucose Needs

Our brains use more energy than any other organ or bodily function. When carb consumption is low, the brain is capable of efficient functions with a minimum amount of glucose (30 grams per day).

The remainder of required energy is provided by ketones. By day 3, our brains have already adapted to operating on 25% ketones[5]. Theoretically this increases to 70% by the seventh day of ketosis.

---

4   "In Silico Evidence for Gluconeogenesis from Fatty Acids in Humans" (2011), http://www.ncbi.nlm.nih.gov/pmc/articles/PMC3140964/

5   "Brain metabolism during short-term starvation in humans" (1994), http://www.ncbi.nlm.nih.gov/pubmed/8263048

Unrelated to weight loss but interesting nonetheless, is the plethora of research projects regarding ketones and brain disease. In an earlier chapter we touched on ketogenic diets for brain trauma and neuro-degenerative disorders. You will find countless research studies on this broad topic. One that is quite interesting and specific is working with omega-3 generated ketones to reduce cognitive deterioration3.

Consider as well the research and latest news reports on the effect of medium-chain fatty acid generated ketones as a prevention and cure for Alzheimer's and ALS. This is most intriguing as coconut oil is the richest source of medium-chain fatty acids and is also a favored fat source in high fat diet communities.

How To Know You're Keto-Adapted (In Ketosis)

We've already discussed that while in ketosis, ketones enter the bloodstream and that only a small amount are excreted in urine, sweat and saliva.

Therefore, the most reliable method is to test with a blood test monitor and ketone strips. Reliable, but also expensive. A monitor may only be $20, but a box of strips are currently priced at 10 for $45 with no market indication of an upcoming decrease.

The best free indication of keto-adaptation is the lack of constant hunger.

I'm serious.

If you were a disciplined and healthy eater before you started this diet you may forget to eat once you become keto-adapted.

If you had been eating a high carb diet before starting this diet, the change is inescapable and unmistakable. You won't be thinking about your next meal shortly after completing the last one. You won't be thinking of a snack after dinner while watching the television, you'll just be enjoying the show.

You can also measure the small percentage of ketones (type: acetoacetate) that are expelled through urine, sweat or saliva. The smell of these ketones are unique and unpleasant. The underlying scent is of acetone with a pungent fruity, and sometimes rancid, tone.

These same ketones can be detected by urine test strips[6] ($22/100 strips); not always reliably, but are far cheaper than the blood test strips. The ultimate range for fat-burning – I've been told and have never gone above this level personally – is within "Trace 5-0.5" and "Small 15-1.5" (the first two color changes on the bottle) using KetoStix by Bayer.

There will only be one type of ketone in your urine and detection is affected by your level of hydration. During this diet you should be drinking sufficient water, plus broth and teas. As such, the presence of ketones could be so faint that a test strip won't register them. On the other side, both exercise and consumption of medium-chain fatty acids (coconut oil) can create a rise in urinary ketone levels.

These strips do not work for everyone, *or* consistently, *or* during all stages of ketosis. However, if they do work for you, you'll probably love using them. It is always pleasant to see progress – in the mirror, by the way your clothes fit, on the scale, by the measuring tape, and with a little stick that you pee on.

If you don't have acetone breath, or stinky urine, or see a color change on the test strip, do not stress about it. Judge your keto-adaptation by the way you feel, by the change in your cravings and hunger levels, and best of all, by weight loss.

---

6   http://www.ketohybrid.com/ketostix

CHAPTER 5

Carbohydrates: Starch, Sugar, and Fiber

Avoid most carbohydrates and you'll naturally lose weight. In full disclosure initial weight loss due to low-carb consumption is attributed to the release of water retention, but that release is the vital first step of shrinking fat cells.

When you're starting out, watching and counting carbs will take up the lion's share of your attention. Empty carbohydrates are found in the strangest of places and in shockingly high numbers. Become familiar with the net carb count of your favorite foods (some are listed in next chapter) and commit to ditching those high-carb foods.

Know Your Food Labels

Check every food label for carbohydrates per serving before purchase. If you're not sure and the product isn't labeled, use your phone to run a search on Google for the product. Better yet, leave the product in the store.

Look for hidden carbs in the ingredients list as well. Sugars and fillers in trace amounts do not have to be calculated or disclosed on nutrition labels. If there's enough hidden carbs, you will not lose weight. (Yet another reason for eating whole, homemade foods.)

While scrutinizing nutrition labels, check the suggested serving size. Some manufacturers will calculate a single serving as a portion of the container – even though we all know the container is too small to share. This tactic might fool some of their customers some of the time, but it won't be fooling you.

Carb Consumption

Vary the vegetables you eat over the course of a week. It keeps your diet interesting while providing a wider range of naturally obtained vitamins and minerals. Ideally your daily carb macro should be spent on fiber-rich vegetables.

The average person will need to keep net carbohydrate intake within 20-35 grams per day to lose weight. However, a glance at the examples below shows the wide variance between two people. It never hurts to check your statistics and work with suggested net carb intake based on macros. We've set up an online tool[7] that allows you to do so. As your weight changes you should revisit this page again, so please bookmark it, favorite it, or share it in your social networks while you're there.

Two examples:

Male, physically demanding job. 6'5", 240 pounds
Currently using 4006 calories per day.
To lose weight he's chosen a 15% reduction in calories = 3405 calories per day.
Macros set at F: 60; C: 10; P: 30
Daily Result: 85.1 grams carb, 255.4 grams protein, 227 grams fat

Female, desk job. 5'11", 205 pounds
Currently using 1978 calories per day.
To lose weight, she's chosen a 20% reduction in calories = 1640 calories per day.
Macros set at F: 65; C: 5; P: 30
Daily Result: 20.5 grams carb, 123 grams protein, 118.4 grams fat

Vegetables

Aside from tubers, we suggest you use *at least half* your carb allowance on vegetables. Try them all. Try them in different ways. Slather them in butter, saute them in lard, and roast them on the grill. Puree them for soups, or pour on the hollandaise. There are as many ways to prepare them as there are vegetables.

---

7   http://www.ketohybrid.com/calculate

In the beginning of your diet, you'll want to handpick a few favorite low carb vegetables. The lower the net carb count, the larger the portion you can have.

Once your body adjusts to not being hungry all the time, and you're eating small portions as a result, move into some of the higher carb vegetables to broaden your range. You'll find a list of vegetables in the next chapter with their net carb value.

Our Favorite Leafy Vegetables

Arugula (0.4/cup) is very low in carbs but an acquired taste. Romaine (0.6/cup) is readily available as organic produce and quite versatile (it even tastes great slightly grilled).

Spinach	vs	Romaine
23	calories	15
79	sodium (mg)	28
558	potassium (mg)	194
3.6	carbohydrate (grams)	2.9
2.2	fiber (grams)	1.3
2.9	protein (grams)	1.4
9377	vitamin a (IU)	7405
28.1	vitamin c (mg)	9.2
99	calcium (mg)	36
2.7	iron (mg)	0.9
0.2	b-6 (mg)	0.1
79	magnesium (mg)	13

The real powerhouse though is spinach (1.0/cup). Fresh spinach lasts longer in your fridge, is delicious hot or cold and ounce for ounce has more nutrition.

Our Favorite Cooked Vegetables

Rapini (0.1/cup) wins hands down. It is practically all fiber but tastes like broccoli (4.4/cup) and cooks in less time. It can be slightly bitter which gives you a great reason to drizzle on garlic-infused olive oil once it is out of the saute pan.

Rapini	vs	Broccoli
22	calories	34
33	sodium (mg)	33
196	potassium (mg)	316
2.8	carbohydrate (grams)	7.0
2.7	fiber (grams)	2.6
3.2	protein (grams)	2.8
2622	vitamin a (IU)	623
20.2	vitamin c (mg)	89.2
108	calcium (mg)	47
2.1	iron (mg)	0.7
0.2	b-6 (mg)	0.2
22	magnesium (mg)	21

We also favor asparagus (3.8/cup), cauliflower (2.9/cup), mushrooms (1.6/cup), summer squash (2.6/cup), and green peppers (4.4/cup). You don't have to stick to our favorites though; there are many other low carb vegetables available.

We Avoid These Vegetables

We use scallions or green onions regularly (4.0/cup), but generally steer clear of other onion varieties (10.0-14.0/cup).

Carrots (7.4/cup) taste too sweet now. Garlic (42.1/cup) – thank goodness we don't ever want to eat a full cup. Corn (25.2/cup) – dangerously genetically modified; not worth the bother. Potatoes (32.1/cup) and sweet potatoes (34.8/cup), beets (13.6/cup), butternut squash (15.0/cup) and fresh peas without the pod (13.6/cup) – all too high for the nutrition they offer.

Sugars

Sugar has only become a real problem for the human race in the last 200 years. It is estimated that the average American eats over 150 pounds of sugar per year. Compare that to 63 pounds in the previous century; 7.5 pounds in the century before that.

Most of us aren't aware of our sugar intake. A popular television doctor suggests that 50 percent of the sugar we eat comes in the form of hidden sugar and high-fructose corn syrup.

Here is a short list of (what the industry considers) healthy foods, even though they contain added sugar:

    100% whole grain bread
    canned soups, sauces and vegetables
    fat-free salad dressing
    granola
    pickles
    protein bars
    pre-packaged oatmeal
    peanut butter
    yogurt

Natural sugars are very high in carbohydrates and have no nutritional value. These include white sugar, brown sugar, honey, fruit sugars and molasses.

Effect of Natural Sugars vs Fructose

Natural sugars are metabolized by our body in a natural way (blood sugar rises, insulin releases, absorption, storage, etc.)

Fructose tricks our bodies and does not stimulate a rise in blood sugar. This is one of the reasons the medical community considered fructose to be a safe additive for so many years.

Only recently have we discovered that fructose isn't harmless at all! Fructose promotes insulin resistance, eventually damaging a body's ability to cope with any type of carbohydrate.

This damage has long-term consequences.

While natural sugars are lacking, fructose is even worse (commonly found in foods as high fructose corn syrup but goes by many other names).

Corn, wheat, potatoes, rice, pasta, legumes and beans that are high in starch should be thought of as sugars in disguise.

Starches contain a high percentage of sugar molecules that your digestive system treats the same way as natural sugar – "let's break it down and send it to the bloodstream!"

Sugar Substitutes

The opinion, distaste, or love for sugar substitutes vary widely. This is one of few topics we (as a mother and daughter) agree to disagree upon. Mom said "Age trumps beauty. I'm writing this section of the book!"

Four Reasons To Dislike Sugar Substitutes

#1 TASTE I have yet to find a sugar substitute that doesn't leave a bitter or chemical aftertaste in my mouth. When Stevia first hit the mainstream marketplace (2000), it was 'acceptable' in taste as long as the sweetness of a dish wasn't the primary factor and the tang of it could be masked behind strong flavors. The manufacturing process of Stevia today has altered it's natural sweetness. If you are going to use it, get the most natural source you can find.

#2 CHEMICAL PROCESSING OR ADDITIVES Like #1, this is a personal opinion, but I am of firm belief that the added chemicals in our foods – whether it be flavoring, dye, hormones, antibiotics, pesticides, those used for extraction or preservatives – are the root cause of inflammation and most illness. As a society – just a few generations past the era of whole and fresh foods being the main staple of our diets – we have grown far too accepting and accustomed to these additives. All mass produced sugar substitutes have undergone some chemical processing or transformation.

#3 NOT ENOUGH RESEARCH We don't have enough research data, nor has enough time passed, to know how sugar substitutes of any type affect our bodies in the long term. To illustrate, we once thought fructose was safe for diabetics because the ingestion of it didn't cause a rise in blood sugar – we now know that it is incredibly unsafe for all of us. We also once thought that aspartame, saccharin, and sucralose were safe (all classified by the US FDA as GRAS, generally regarded as safe) – only to discover decades later that they are or might be responsible for many ills; including but not limited to cancer, DNA damage, and intestinal problems.

#4 CRAVINGS Who doesn't enjoy a sweet treat? The trouble is they're addictive and you pay for the indulgence with annoying cravings for days after. Sugar substitutes create the same response in our bodies. When you break the sweet habit, you not only stop the incessant cravings but your taste buds change. You begin to notice the subtle sweetness in natural and healthy foods. As an example, I thinly sliced carrots for our KetoHybrid Matzo Ball soup last week and found them to be too sweet. Lose the sweet tooth and an entire new world of flavors becomes available.

Safest Sugar Substitutes In Order of Acceptability

Personal distaste of sweeteners aside, we're not so far into eating the KetoHybrid way that we've forgotten how hard it is to give up sweet snacks.

Denying yourself too often and for too long is a common reason for complete diet abandonment.

Will a handful of berries quell your craving? If so, that natural route is the healthiest possible way to treat yourself.

If not – and because we don't want you to ditch your diet over such a silly thing as sugar – the list below contains some of the safest, natural, and low carb sweeteners available. Please only use them in moderation or you'll never break your sweet attraction.

You'll find recipes for sweet baked goods in a latter chapter of this book. We have left it to you to decide which sweetener, if any, you want to use. We have made some of the mug cakes without any added sweetener – other than berries or by adding real whipped cream as a topping – and they can quiet cravings and nix the feeling of deprivation.

Your taste buds will start registering the natural sweetness of foods in about 4 weeks. Almonds, carrots, limes and peas all taste naturally sweet to me now.

Stevia

An all natural, calorie free herb, commonly found as a manufactured liquid or powder extract. The extract is 200+ times sweeter than sugar and hasn't yet been associated with health-robbing side effects.

In the last 15 years, the use of Stevia in sugar substitute blends and pre-packaged foods has increased. Although these blends and foods appear healthy because they contain an all natural, low calorie sweetener, those pre-packaged foods often contain other additives that you won't want in your body.

The Stevia plant can be grown and harvested, or purchased as an organic, dry, food additive. Drops that are 100% Stevia are more versatile for baking or sweetening drinks.

Monk Fruit (Lo Han) Powder

Monk Fruit powder is comparable to Stevia; 300 times sweeter than sugar, but without the bitter aftertaste. These powders are often mixed with inulin (see below). Monk Fruit powder is very expensive but, like Stevia, you won't be using much of it at a time.

Sugar Alcohols

Also called polyols, these sugar substitutes are extracted from plants and/or manufactured from starches. These inlcude Erythritol, Sorbitol and Xylitol to name but a few.

Sugar alcohols are made by extracting sugars from plants (traditionally fruit, but are now commonly made from corn, wheat, and hardwood). Extracted sugar is mixed with water, then fermented, filtered, crystallized, and dried. The end result are white crystals, granules or powder.

Sugar alcohols sound promising. They are zero-to-low calorie, low carb, and made from natural sources. The manufacturing process however, is not natural.

These alcohols have been in existence since the late 1800's, but they haven't been widely used and since their initial discovery we've changed the creation/extraction process. All of this should cause some pause. Will sugar alcohols be discovered as unsafe as saccharin and other harmful sugar substitutes; 20 years after we've all consumed them to excess?

In large quantities sugar alcohols may cause nausea and diarrhea.

Erythritol serves up 0.2 calories per gram and is used in many sugar substitute blends. Approximately 90% of Erythritol is excreted by the body, unchanged, with no effect on blood glucose. This sugar alcohol is 60-70% as sweet as sugar and costs four times the price.

Mannitol (aka manna sugar or mannite) serves up 1.5 calories per gram and also does not affect blood sugar. Mannitol's primary source was the ash tree. It is 60% as sweet as sugar and costs approximately 10 times the price.

Xylitol serves up 2.5 calories per gram and is as sweet as sugar. Xylitol's original primary source was the birch tree. It is highly toxic to dogs and is about four times the price of sugar.

Sorbitol serves up 2.5 calories per gram and is 60% as sweet as sugar. It is mostly derived from corn syrups.

Inulin

Inulin is a naturally occurring dietary fiber made from the chicory root. It contains some calories and has a mild effect on blood sugar – 57 calories per ounce and 2.3 net carbs respectively. As one of North America's most popular sugar substitutes, inulin is also derived from jicama, bananas, onions, and Jerusalem artichokes. Inulin-based sweeteners are not stable at temperatures over 245°F/120°C which rule them out for use in baked goods.

Flours

Although traditional wheat flour is impossible to perfectly replace, alternatives exist for specific needs.

You won't need all of the following ingredients to make the recipes in this book, nor do you need to become familiar with them all. Almond flour, coconut flour, golden flax and psyllium are our favorites for baking – which we do less and less every month.

All of the items below can be purchased at a bulk food store, health food store, health aisle of large grocery stores, or online.

Flour Substitutes

Almond Flour, nothing more than ground almonds really, can be used for baking. The flour is so versatile, satisfying, and health-filled it is easy to forget that while it is low in carbs, it is high in calories. The flour comes in two varieties – normal and blanched. I don't find much difference in the flavor but the blanched makes a consistently lighter (color) baked good. One cup of almond flour contains approximately 90 average size almonds. (9 net carbs per cup)

Basan (Chickpea Flour) is not exactly diet friendly, but in very small quantities it is a nice flour for blending when you need to add in a smooth texture. (43 net carbs per cup)

Coconut Flour, is another highly nutritious flour that fits the low carb high fat lifestyle. It is high in fiber but it seldom stands alone and does well in a recipe. Great for adding bulk and smoothing out texture, but it can be heavy in the pan and on the tongue. Mixing with other flours and/or ample eggs makes it more versatile. (6 net carbs per ounce or 2 tbsp)

Flax Seeds (aka Ground Flax, Flax Seed Meal), is highly nutritious and high in fiber. Readily available in two different types – regular and golden. Both are low in carbs and low in taste (great for bulking up baked goods without masking other flavors). The golden variety is softer and airier than standard flax (a dark brown in color). If you substitute regular ground in recipes that call for golden, you end up with a tougher and heavier, end product. (3 net carbs per cup)

Guar Gum, is used in small quantities as a binder in baked goods. Interchangeable with Xanthan Gum. May cause stomach discomfort. (0.0 net carbs)

Psyllium (aka Psyllium Husks) are available as a ground seed or a powder. Both husks and powder can replace Xanthum or Guar Gum in any recipe. With equal amounts of water and a little time (15-20 minutes) psyllium turns gelatinous, elastic – as you'd like gluten to behave in fact. It is also a great bulking agent or additive. (3 net carbs per ounce)

Vital Wheat Gluten is made from the protein part of the wheat and is carb. Very binding, so use in very small amounts when you need a little gluten to thicken sauces, make gravy, or add some springiness to your baked goods. High in protein. (4 grams carbs per ounce)

Wheat Bran is low carb but it cannot be used as a replacement for another 'flour'. It does function as a bulking additive and when toasted lends a nutty flavor to finished loaves or muffins. It does have a tendency to dry out the finished product so only supplement recipes in small quantities (5-7%) and/or soak the bran first for 20 minutes in an equal amount of warm water. (12 net carbs per cup)

Xanthan Gum, is used in small quantities as a binder in baked goods. Interchangeable with Guar Gum. May cause stomach discomfort. (0.0 net carbs)

CHAPTER 6

Fats

Keeping fat intake high presents a challenge for many of us. For years we've been conditioned to dislike fats based on the premise of "eat fat and you'll get fat"; which simply isn't true.

Even when you've poured over the research and decided to let more healthy fats into your diet, it still takes some time for your taste buds to accept that large gobs of butter and ounces of drizzled olive oil are acceptable.

Eating nuts make adding fats to your diet, easy. The higher the fat content, the better. (Go easy in the beginning. If you're not used to them, they can cause gut inflammation.)

Buy fatty cuts or well-marbled meat and don't be afraid to eat the fat. The healthiest fats come from natural, grass-fed, or organically raised animals. I do not suggest eating the fat of an animal from a large scale, commercial farm. Most animals, humans included, store toxins in fat cells.

Load on the sauces. Hollandaise and mayonnaise are two high fat sauces that are completely acceptable on this diet.

Drizzle on the virgin olive oil. Buy only the best and add it to your meat and vegetables after cooking. Having a few bottles of herb-infused oils on hand for drizzling keeps dinners interesting. Garlic-infused oil is a fantastic way to add garlic taste to your meal without adding a lot of extra carbohydrates. Rosemary infused oil is another favorite in our house.

Whipping cream makes everything taste better. Use heavy cream in your coffee. Make an Alfredo sauce for vegetables or zucchini noodles – fantastic!

Cook your foods in virgin coconut oil, tallow or lard. All three can withstand the high temperatures required in cooking. Coconut oil can also replace butter, shortening, or lard in most recipes.

All seed and nut oils (coconut, flax, grape, olive, sesame, etc.) should be virgin grade and either cold pressed or expeller pressed. The first extraction (extra virgin) preserves all beneficial vitamins and flavor of the oil. Subsequent extractions (virgin) are less beneficial but still trump other oils in nutrition and taste.

Coconut oil is high in medium-chain fatty acids and is the quickest, easiest form of energy for your keto-adapted metabolism. If you like coconut oil eat a teaspoonful right out of the jar to quiet hunger while providing instant clarity and (almost instant) energy.

Make your own bacon and keep the lard to use for warm salad dressings, to saute vegetables or for frying eggs. Lard also has a high smoke point, meaning you can cook it at high temperatures with minimal risk of carcinogens. If you don't cook bacon but want lard, buy fresh pork fat and render it at home (2 hours on low in the slow cooker). It is economical and you can be certain of quality control.

Fats to Eat, Fats to Avoid

Eat butter, ghee, avocado oil, virgin olive oil, virgin coconut oil, flax seed oil, sesame seed oil, grape seed oil, and any virgin nut oil that interests you or that your budget allows.

Steer clear of other oils as the industry makes a mess of them in the manufacturing process.

Commercial and manufactured oils are to be thanked for making so many of us sick. Hydrogenated or partially hydrogenated oils contain trans fats which cause multiple health problems. Readily available vegetable-based cooking oils are high in Omega 6s and made in such large quantities that low quality cannot be detected. Every time you reach for a gallon of oil, envision the large vat it came from – potentially being mixed with rancid oils to cut profit losses, and partially hydrogenating for a longer shelf life (but not labelled as such). Furthermore the extraction – heat or chemical – all but ruins any nutritional value. For the record, these are the same oils your favorite fast food restaurants are using.

For all the reasons in the previous paragraph, do not buy any food products that have oils listed in the ingredients. Over processed and rancid oils that don't make it to the jug are easily disguised by other ingredients and flavors in prepared foods. KetoHybrid is as focused on quality control as it is about balancing macros.

Margarine is out. Even if it says heart-healthy or contains virgin oils.

Commercially prepared mayonnaise is out. Even if the label says "made with olive oil". The two top brands of olive oil mayonnaise actually contain 3 types of oils plus sugar in the ingredients. (I'll show you how to make mayonnaise quickly, healthfully and easily in the chapter on sauces.)

Smoke Points of Fats & Oils

Knowing your oil's smoke point is invaluable. This is the temperature at which an oil breaks down when heat is applied. The oil becomes toxic, which can also happen as a result of repeatedly heating an oil.

You won't be able to tell by the taste. You won't even feel ill. With continued abuse however, you will compromise your immunity and the damage might be irreversible. Substances found in foods cooked in or with oils that have reached their smoke point include peroxides, aldehydes, and hydroperoxides.

Oils with a low smoke point are best used as salad dressings or drizzling over food after the cooking process.

Purchase and use the correct fats and oils based on the temperature required during cooking.

- Frying foods require temperatures of 320-460°F, 160-240°C.
- Sauteing or cooking in a wok will be slightly higher.
- Roasting and baking; the internal temperature of the food within.

Smoke Points

Almond Oil	*430°F	221°C
Avocado Oil	520°F	271°C
Butter (grass fed)	302°F	150°C
Cashew Oil	*	
Chia Oil	*	
Chicken Fat	375°F	190°C
Coconut Oil	350°F	177°C
Coconut Oil (refined)	450°F	232°C
Duck Fat	375°F	190°C
Flax Seed Oil	*	
Ghee	482°F	250°C
Goat Fat	370°F	188°C
Goose Fat	375°F	190°C
Grapeseed Oil	*	
Hazelnut Oil	430°F	221°C
Hemp Seed Oil	*	
Lard	394°F	201°C
Macadamia Nut Oil	390°F	200°C
Virgin Olive Oil	420°F	215°C
Olive Oil, Extra Virgin	406°F	207°C
Palm Oil	446°F	230°C
Pecan Oil	**	
Pine Nut Oil	**	
Pistachio Oil	*	
Sesame Seed Oil	*	
Tallow	420°F	220°C
Walnut Oil, unrefined	320°F	160°C
Walnut Oil, semi-refined	400°F	204°C

* Flavorful; perfect for dressings or drizzling. Keep refrigerated. Not suitable for cooking with 15% or higher amounts of Poly-Unsaturated Fatty Acids (PUFAs) which, when oxidized by heat or oxygen, form higher amounts of toxic peroxides which may cause cellular damage.

** No smoke point information available at this time but do contain high levels of PUFAs.

CHAPTER 7

Proteins

We have such a wide variety of protein sources to choose from – you'll never be bored! You do need to be picky about your proteins though, ensuring they only come from the best sources and free from harmful handling or manufacturing processes.

If you have land and the inclination, grow your own food. Cows, pigs and chickens aren't terribly time consuming. Many people do this while managing full-time jobs outside of the home. We did it all on our little hobby farm for years.

All of these changes will increase your grocery budget by 15-20% for the first month, but there's simply no way around it. If you follow our suggestions to perfection, you will gain that money back by not grabbing a muffin at the drive-through or buying lunch at the office. A $5 breakfast and $10 lunch equates to $75/week. At 50 weeks per annum, that's $3,750 you'll save!

Trust us on this. When you are fully keto-adapted your grocery budget returns to a reasonable amount. You will be getting more nutrition in every bite, you'll be eating and wasting less, and you'll save money. Cookies, breads, convenience or processed foods are actually quite expensive!

Red Meat: Beef, Pork, Wild Game

Buy organic, grass fed or pasture raised products only. This specialty food is now available in most grocery stores, but you can save money by getting to know your local butcher.

A well managed, privately-owned butcher shop knows where their product comes from. They can help you find the best meat, grown by the best practices. Our little butcher shop has our phone number in their book; whenever they receive a pastured animal they call for an order. Your butcher should do the same.

If you have the time, take a country drive and shake hands with a few farmers. Small farms that don't mind the intrusion will have signs posted at the end of their driveway. You can also check in at a livestock supply store for contact numbers or pick them off the store's bulletin boards. Commit to purchasing a side of beef or a pig from the farmer when they're ready to slaughter – you'll need a freezer, but you'll save money while ensuring quality.

You may have some emotional unrest over this, that's normal. We are all quite disconnected from our food. We can't handle the thought of the cow seen lazing in the field one week, laying across our plate the next. It's unsettling. There is merit – whether you are on the KetoHybrid diet or not – in knowing where your food comes from, how it was raised, and what it was fed or injected with. There is so much wrong with commercial meat packers, feed lots, and up-scaled farms.

Know your food. Don't consume misery.

Poultry & Eggs

The advice above stands for all poultry. Raise your own poultry, commit to a farmer's stock, or talk to your local butcher. If your only option is the grocery store, choose organic. Yes you'll be paying more and getting lesser volume, but the nutrition and flavor justify the cost.

FREE RANGE: Hens are allowed out of doors, scratching in the dirt and eating bugs – they produce the best quality egg.

FREE RUN: Hens are allowed to move about in a barn or their enclosure – they produce a good quality egg.

COMMERCIALLY-HARVESTED: Hens live miserable lives in tiny cages – eggs are pale and thin, and two weeks old by the time you get them.

Free range or free run eggs are also wise investments. We went through a lot of eggs when we started this diet and since the farm was an hour's drive we'd buy 7-8 dozen at a time. Fresh eggs from the farm, especially if they are unwashed, will stay fresh for over a month.

Fish & Shellfish

All fish and shellfish is acceptable with the exception of pickled, creamed, or artificial varieties. We stay away from farmed fish, having watched too much footage of disgusting fish farm practices.

Fish

Canned wild fish is occasionally acceptable but you might have to do a little research to find an additive-free, BPA-free, soy free (yes, that seems odd but many large packers have soy in the cans), low mercury, and sustainably caught brands. Alaskan wild salmon is currently the best bet for canned salmon (with the same conditions of the can as for tuna).

Firm Fleshed Fish (grill)
Arctic Char
Grouper
Halibut
Haddock
Mahi Mahi
Marlin
Monkfish
Red Snapper
Salmon
Swordfish
Tuna

Small Fish (snacks)
Anchovies
Herring
Mackerel
Sardines
Smelt

Fillets (pan fry or bake)
Bass (all types)
Branzini
Catfish
Flounder
Perch
Pickerel/Walleye
Pike
Sole
Trout (all types)

Mild Flavored and Versatile
Cod
Crappie
Fluke
Mullet
Orange Roughy
Shad
Tilapia
Whitefish

Shellfish & Seafood

Shrimp, mussels and lobster are all best purchased fresh at a fish market where you can specifically request ocean harvested shellfish – they will be expensive but are superior in quality. Most of our shellfish supply is farmed, generally in less than perfect conditions, and they do not eat a natural diet. There is a little saving grace though, shellfish are low in fat and highly resistant to heavy metal toxins.

Scallops should be purchased as dry packed, or frozen and vacuum-sealed. Even if you're on the coast, request dry scallops only. Wet scallops float in a brine that contains sodium tripolyphosphate, yet another preservative that has been labeled GRAS by the FDA.

- Abalone
- Clams
- Conch
- Crabs (incl. Softshell)
- Crawfish/Crayfish
- Cuttlefish
- Krill
- Langoustines
- Lobster
- Mussels
- Octopus
- Oysters
- Prawns
- Roe (Lobster/Crab/Shrimp/Prawn)
- Sea Cucumbers
- Sea Snails (inc. Periwinkle)
- Sea Urchins
- Scallops
- Shrimp
  (including Squilla Mantis)
- Squid

CHAPTER 8

Nuts & Seeds

Nuts add versatility, protein and fats to recipes as well as being one of the perfect low-carb snacks. They are easy to overeat so limit your intake to 2-3 ounces per day if weight loss is your goal. Pre-roasted nuts may contain added oil, salt, sugar, or curing chemicals.

Seeds offer preventative health benefits but some smaller varieties (flax, sesame and un-hulled hemp) must be ground so your body can absorb the nutrition.

Chia seeds (Salvia hispanica) are soft shelled and literally melt in your mouth. As such your body easily absorbs the protein and potassium this seed contains. Those unique qualities of chia also make it incredibly versatile in the kitchen. In this book we use it to make jam but it also makes great low carb puddings and thickens gravy.

Preparing & Storing Nuts

Nuts contain phytic acid and a high percentage of enzyme inhibitors which can make them hard on your digestive system. If you have tummy trouble (a heavy feeling) after snacking on a few nuts you might want to try soaking them[8]. Doing so neutralizes those pesky enzymes, allows proper digestion and ensures that you are getting full nutrition from the nuts you eat.

Refrigerate all nuts and seeds whether they are raw or roasted. Except for cashews you can hull and roast your own nuts (15 minutes in a 350°F degree oven on a baking sheet).

8   How to soak nuts. www.KetoHybrid.com/nuts

Nut Butters & More

Nuts and seeds also make delicious butters, oils, milks, and flours. Grind roasted nuts in a food processor until the butter reaches desired consistency, add a teaspoon of coconut butter per cup of nuts to make it smoother. A pinch of salt per cup may heighten the flavor.

The Perils of Peanuts & Peanut Butter

Peanuts are not an allowable nut. Peanuts are legumes and are not recommended. If commercially prepared peanut butter is a staple in your cupboard take a look at the label and see what you've been eating. Unhealthy oils, sugars, and salt - all unnecessary additives. I've never understood the reasoning for all those additives; all-natural peanut butter has the same shelf life as commercially prepared peanut butter.

Rants aside, peanut butter is not healthy. if you can't live without it, try replacing it with a true nut butter found in health food stores. Almond, hazelnut, cashew and pecan butters are delicious and you can make your own to save money.

CHAPTER 9

Beverages

It is far too easy to drink your carbs, overload the calories, and ingest a bunch of chemicals in the process. A big change in drinking habits could result in a big change on the scales over the span of a few months.

Our low carb side warns you away from milk, fruit juices and sodas. The Paleo-influenced side goes ballistic thinking about the chemicals in diet sodas and flavored waters.

There is no relief in Keto diets either – you're limited to water, herbal teas, a morning coffee or two, and perhaps a little wine or alcohol.

Water

Water, when we were on the farm, was a deliciously viable option. Our well was fed by a cold spring, coming right off mountains of the Canadian Shield. This was the only place we ever drank water from the tap; never filtered, never treated.

Today Veronica lives in a large city and I live in a nearby town. Our water is treated by our municipalities and neither smells nor tastes like anything you'd want to swallow. The earth-loving side of us won't buy into bottled water.

So what do we do? We filter the heck out of it. Veronica filters her water with a tabletop pitcher and I use a reverse-osmosis under-counter unit. These make water palatable, but here's how we make it tasty:

- Throw a few frozen raspberries in your glass. Incredible how much 2-3 berries can alter the flavor of an entire glass.

- Add a few sprigs of fresh mint. For even more variety, grow some chocolate mint or spearmint in a little pot on your kitchen counter.
- A tiny squeeze of a lemon, lime or orange adds a negligible amount of carbs and calories and tastes great.
- Make a pot of herbal tea and refrigerate it. Cold herbal teas are properly called tisanes. Who knew they had such a fancy name? You can make them with fresh ginger, your favorite blend of chai spices (cinnamon, cloves and cardamom), or even with your own favorite herbal tea bags.

Washing Away The Toxins

Once you've made the switch to better eating habits your body begins to rid itself of accumulated toxins through your urine and sweat glands. This is the detox phase; generally lasting seven days but the cleansing could carry on for many weeks.

Water consumption is the most supportive way to help your body do its job. Recommended water intake is 8-12 eight ounce glasses per day. If you're a larger person, working hard and sweating a lot, you may need more.

Can you overdo it with water? Absolutely. While every glass consumed is a gift, there is a point when all that water is no longer effective and may cause undue stress. This happens when electrolytes and sodium are unbalanced or when the dieter isn't getting enough sleep because they're up 3-4 times in the night to urinate.

Here is my suggestion. Drink water through the day at the recommended rate with adjustments for your size, the climate and your activity. Throughout the day, watch the color of your urine. If your urine runs clear, lay off water intake for at least an hour. Also refrain from drinking water two hours before bed.

Alcoholic Beverages

Dry wines in moderation have been proven to be beneficial. If you enjoy it, you should continue to; keeping in mind every ounce will contain about 1 net carb; standard serving size for wine is five ounces.

The sweeter the wine, the more carbs and calories inside. White wine is almost as beneficial to health as red. Dry champagnes or sparkling whites are generally 70% lower in carbs than other wines but have almost as many calories.

In the past, beer drinkers would need to consider imbibing in their favorite beverage, a cheat. Today there are many low carb varieties to choose from and most of them are classified as light beers. Ounce for ounce beer is slightly higher in carbs than wine; a double-edged sword since you're not likely to find a 5 ounce bottle (beer usually arrives in a 12 ounce bottle so you could be drinking up to 18 net carbs even in a light beer).

At the end of hot summer's day, sitting back with an ice cold Canadian beer on the deck is pure heaven, but have you ever looked at the ingredient label? No? That's because there isn't one.

In the United States and in Canada breweries are exempt from the standard requirement of listing ingredients on the label. That should concern you.

Commercial breweries use (some or all) of the following ingredients in the creation of beer: GMO corn and corn syrup; high fructose corn syrup; GMO dextrose; GMO rice (yes, rice); propylene glycol (please read my warning about food flavorings in the desserts section and how small doses of propylene glycol is known for preventing weight loss); fish bladder; caramel coloring; formaldehyde; MSG; dyes; BPA and more.

Finally we come to straight, non-flavored alcohol. Vodka, gin, scotch and the like are practically carb free but even just an ounce of alcohol will have an effect on your blood sugar. Many of us (but not everyone) will get kicked right out of ketosis when having just a few shots of alcohol.

CHAPTER 10

Herbs and Spices

Take an average meal of meat or eggs and vegetables, and make it exquisite with just a few herbs and spices.

Fresh chopped herbs bring delicious flavors to soups and stews when added right before serving.

Experiment by coarsely chopping basil, borage, chicory, fennel, oregano, parsley or watercress and add them to your salad greens.

In the last few years studies have shown that grilled meats might increase cancer risk (some people, some cancers). Studies are also showing that marinating or mixing meats with rosemary and/or other herbs reduce the risk significantly[9].

As always, fresh and organic is best, but keep your cupboards stocked with dried herbs and spices as well. Herbs are delicate and often over-sprayed with pesticides. While you're not consuming large quantities of them, if we're going to be pristine in our consumption we might as well consider every bite.

If you buy fresh herbs at the grocery store, immediately remove the metal tie or rubber band at the base, trim 1/4" off the stem and keep your herbs upright in a tall glass with 1" water. We use herb keepers during the winter months as they protect delicate leaves while providing water at the roots. You can also store them, short term, in a slightly damp paper towel in your crisper. Wash herbs before use – not before storage.

---

9   "Effect of marinades on the formation of heterocyclic amines in grilled beef steaks," (2008), http://www.ncbi.nlm.nih.gov/pubmed/19241593

If you are cooking for a large family, you'll use your herbs up before they go bad. Our family is tiny so we wash, mince and freeze half of every bundle we buy. Adding a little olive oil to the mince helps to protect flavors from freezer burn. Frozen herbs are perfect for soups, sauces, salad dressings and marinades.

Dried spices and herbs should be kept in a cool, dark cupboard. Dried spice blends (i.e. steak rubs, lemon pepper), pickled enhancers (i.e. prepared horseradish), and tubed herb pastes may contain additives you don't want in your mouth.

You can make your own curry, garam masala, poultry seasoning, Italian herb blends, steak rubs and more at home and to your taste. Continue to read your labels on every product, no matter how small. (Watch for sugars, dextrose, oils, salts, and chemicals in every wet-packed product.)

Using and Knowing Herbs and Spices

Everyone has their own favorite spices. Experiment and try your favorites with any dish.

Allspice, for example, is traditionally it is used in pumpkin pies and Jamaican meat stews – but why not try it on vegetables before roasting or grilling? If it pairs well with pumpkin, it may just do the same with other squash such as zucchini.

A pepper grinder is one of the nicest gifts you can give yourself. Freshly ground peppercorns are out of this world! If you already have one, you can spoil yourself instead with a spice grinder (often sold as coffee bean grinders). They cost less than $20 and come in handy when making your own spice blends, grinding flax seeds, or chopping nuts.

If you buy a pepper grinder - get two and use the other for Himalayan Pink Salt[10]. Purchase granules instead of ground salt for your new grinder. You'll feel like a true chef!

Allspice: Deep pungent, slightly peppery flavor. Very similar to cloves in flavor and usage. Used in baking (sweets), sauces and salsas, and in slow cooked stews.

---

10 "Why Pink Salt?" www.KetoHybrid.com/pinksalt

Basil: Robust flavor that is slightly licorice, slightly mint, slightly woodsy. The main flavor in pesto. Used in many traditional pasta sauces and salad dressings. Try it in your vegetable saute pan with a little butter.

Bay Leaf: Mellow, woodsy flavor. Usually a background spice or one that helps blend other spices within a recipe. A standard in soups and sauces.

Caraway Seed: Slightly licorice flavored. You've noticed the flavor in rye bread and sauerkraut. Great on roast vegetables and in salad dressings.

Cardamom: Associated mostly with Indian cuisine. One of the prominent flavors in Chai tea. Pairs great with clove and cinnamon. Highly aromatic.

Cayenne Pepper: Made from ground red chili peppers. A sweeter heat than freshly chopped hot peppers. Used in soups and meat dishes. Try it in your salad dressing. This is one to love as it boosts metabolism.

Chervil (herb): A delicate herb that loses almost all flavor when dried or over-cooked. Buy it fresh and in season and add it at the end of the cooking process only. Lightly anise flavored. Chervil is one of the herbs from the famous French "fines herbes" blend.

Cinnamon: Used in both savory and sweet recipes. Also known to boost metabolism.

Cloves: Often used with cinnamon. Most often found in baking. Sweet and warm. Often seen in ham roast or apple recipes. One of the flavors used in curry.

Coriander: These are the dried seeds from the cilantro plant. A similar flavor to fresh cilantro, but different enough to make a distinction. Sometimes interchangeable with cilantro. Lemony flavor. Great in salsas and chutneys. Great when paired with chicken or pork. Found in Indian cuisine and Mexican dishes. Used in curry and in garam masala.

Cumin: Uniquely smoky and earthy flavors. Pungent and powerful. Draws out the slight sweetness of a recipe. Great with vegetables, fish, stews and salad dressings. You may have tasted it in a falafal or couscous. Paired with cauliflower or eggplant it is exquisite. Use sparingly until you fall in love with it.

Dill: A light and feathery herb that loses most of it's flavor in drying. Used most often with pickling, fish, and in some delicate sauces.

Fennel Seed: Similar to caraway but lightly sweet. Excellent with fish, vegetables and in salad dressings.

Fenugreek: Smells sweet when it's cooking but has a burnt sugar taste that is a little on the bitter side. Medicinally it is used to balance estrogen. Note: In some cultures it is believed to facilitate weight gain.

Garlic Powder: Made from dried garlic. Easy to keep and cheap to buy.

Gochugaru/Kochugaru: Made from sun-dried chili peppers. A Korean spice that is hot, sweet, and slightly smoky all at the same time.

Mace: Comes from the same plant as nutmeg and is similar in taste. Often used in stews and homemade sausages.

Marjoram: Both woodsy and floral tones, but delicate. Commonly used in sauces, salad dressings and marinades. Pairs well with sage and rosemary. Wonderful in roasted dishes.

Mint: Intense flavor that goes with nearly everything from chicken to chocolate.

Nutmeg: A warm spice. Delicious when used with baked goods but also found in savory meals.

Oregano: Slight lemon flavor. A strong herb that retains most of it's power in dried form. Used in many sauces, especially in Mexican and Mediterranean cuisine. Great paired with basil or in a salad dressing.

Paprika: A spice suited for most savory dishes. Adds a slightly sweet note and provides an earthy red color.

Pepper: Black pepper is the most common, but white, green and pink pepper each have slightly different flavors and provide variation.

Rosemary: Very strong pine scent and flavor. A standard in poultry seasoning. Also good with baked egg dishes and grilled meats. Proven to bind with and nullify cancer-causing HCAs - the result of grilling meat.

Saffron: In a class all of it's own. Saffron is expensive to harvest but unmistakable in taste. Slightly floral, very yellow. Use moderately.

Sage: Another standard in poultry cooking. Slightly lemon, slightly pine.

Smoked Paprika: Made from smoked red peppers and keeps both the sweet of the pepper with the rich smokey flavor. Great in any savory dish.

Star Anise: Licorice flavor, sometimes used in soups and sauces.

Summer Savory: Similar to thyme but slightly peppery. You may have tasted in poultry bread stuffing (dressing). Best used in meat dishes.

Tarragon: Reminiscent of both rosemary and anise. Great to pair with seafood, eggs, any tomato based recipe and in salad dressings.

Turmeric: A subtle taste but adds a big burst of yellow color to dishes. Mild earthy tones.

Thyme: Earthy, woodsy herb. Also a standard in poultry seasoning.

CHAPTER 11

Foods to Avoid

Now that you've seen all the delicious foods you can enjoy, let's get to the foods that need to be off your list.

Some are listed due to their high carb count. Others are to be avoided because they are generally over-processed or are likely to be genetically modified foods. Should you require clarification on any of these items, do not hesitate to send a note via the website.

Bacon or ham or any meat cured with sugar – Bacon is so easy to make at home – no special equipment needed and we've included the recipe in the chapter on meats.

Breaded, battered, coated, marinated, or rubbed. (You can do all of these things at home in a healthier way.)

Breads – except for the recipes in this book or comparable low carb bread recipes.

Cheese "Products" – food that isn't really cheese, but calls itself cheese. Eat real cheese.

Condiments and Salad Dressings – nearly every condiment is loaded with bad oils, added sugars or unnecessary chemicals.

We buy Worchestershire and soy sauce because we haven't figured out how to make it ourselves. If you can't find organic soy sauce, source out some tamari sauce. Tamari is a little thicker (you'll use less) and it has less chance of being tainted by GMO soy or wheat.

We also buy horseradish – mostly because we don't eat much of it often.

Please don't eat commercially prepared ketchup – one look at the label will tell you why.

Lately we've been buying ground mustard to mix up as we need it.

You can make most of your own condiments, easily and in under 5 minutes. You'll find some recipes to get you started in a later chapter of this book.

Corn – not fresh, not ground into flour, not oil. Maybe if you grow it yourself, as a treat.

Grains – and grain flours including wheat, quinoa, amaranth, buckwheat, spelt, rye, sorghum, and oats. We do include one wheat flour recipe that is low carb and for occasional use.

Legumes – some are named beans and some named peas. Understanding which is a legume and which is not can be tricky. Peanuts are a legume – not a nut, and not recommended. Chickpeas are a legume – not a pea and not recommended. Soy beans are also legumes...

Let's make this easier. Avoid any food with the words beans or peas, other than the occasional green beans and snow peas (these are both high in fiber and low in carbs averaging 4 net grams per cup).

Legumes aren't the health food darling that everyone gives them credit for. They lose most of their nutrition during the cooking process and the minerals that are left behind are blocked by the phytates they contain. They may be beneficial due to the high protein level, but they also contain protease inhibitors (which do everything they can to prevent your body from absorbing that protein).

Legumes can cause hormone troubles, stomach troubles and intestinal troubles. For a *health food*, they really aren't worth the trouble.

Milk – is very high in carbs (plus a long list of other reasons why you wouldn't want to, and don't need to, drink it). If you like milk in your tea, switch to black – it's an easy transition. If you drink milk in your coffee, switch to a high fat cream – it tastes better and it has fewer carbs!

Pasta – pasta is made from grains. Find suggestions for replacing pasta in the recipes section.

Peanuts and peanut butter – peanuts are a legume. See legumes above.

Potatoes – potatoes are off the list, but we have a great faux mashed potato recipe that we know you'll love.

Pre-made, prepared, packaged foods – ready to eat, pre-battered, meal in a box, pre-mixed, just add water; all of it is to be avoided.

Rice – white, brown, wild or otherwise. Replace it with riced cauliflower. You won't notice the difference.

Soy – wouldn't touch it (not milk, flour, or oil) unless it was organic and labeled as non-GMO and only in tofu form. Unfortunately over 90% of soy grown in the USA is GMO. Good organic soy sauce is still made in Japan and aged appropriately.

CHAPTER 12

Carb Counts of Common Foods

This list is for informational use only.

This is not a list of suggested foods.

While we have made every effort to ensure the items are correct in their net carb count, they can vary between manufacturers, growing seasons, or moisture levels.

You may not find your favorite foods or cooking ingredients within this list, but most can be found with a quick search from Google. If you really want to know what's in your food – including calories, cholesterol, sodium, fiber, protein and complete carbohydrates, you would benefit from a book on food counts. We have reviewed a few of them[11].

The list does include all ingredients in KetoHybrid's recipes and some that we guessed you might consider using as substitutes.

Keeping a list like this handy will help you if you ever feel like cheating or quitting altogether. Now that you know the harmful long-term effects of over-carbing, and the health benefits of eating high quality fats, you will never look at food the same way again. When we first started counting carbs, we were shocked at the number of empty carbohydrates in our old diets. We also learned of alternatives to our favorites just by browsing lists like the one below.

Please help us, help each other – if you believe you have found an error please let us know by sending an email to veronica@ketohybrid.com.

---

11 http://www.KetoHybrid.com/food-counts

Beverages

Almond Milk, Plain, Unsweetened	1 cup	1.0
Beer, Nonalcoholic	12 oz	14.1
Bourbon, Gin, Rum, Scotch and Vodka	1 oz	0.0
Carrot Juice	1 cup	20.0
Champagne	4 oz	8.0-12.0
Clam & Tomato Juice	1 cup	28.0
Club Soda	12 oz	0.0
Coconut Milk, canned	1 cup	4.0-6.4
Coconut Milk, Plain	1 cup	7.0
Coconut Milk, Unsweetened	1 cup	1.0
Coconut Water, Fresh	1 cup	6.3
Coffee, black, brewed	1 cup	0.0
Coffee, with 1 T cream		0.4
Coffee, with 1 T milk		0.7
Energy Drinks 1 cup		27.0-30.0
Gatorade 1 cup		15.7
Iced Tea Green, unsweetened	1 cup	0.0
Iced Tea, lemon flavored	1 cup	22.0
Sodas and Tonic Water	12 oz	32.0-42.0
Soy Milk, Plain, Unsweetened	1 cup	2.0
Starbucks Caffè Latte w/ Whole Milk	12 oz	14.0
Starbucks Mocha Frappuccino	12 oz	38.3
Tea, brewed black	1 cup	0.0
Tea, with 1 T milk	1 cup	0.7
Tea, with 1 T cream	1 cup	0.4
Tomato / Vegetable Juice	1 cup	8.0-9.0
Wine, Rose	4 oz	0.6
Wine, Red / White	4 oz	2.2-3.0

Breads

Melba Toast, 1 piece	5 g	4.0
Pita, white	6 1/2"	32.0
Saltine Crackers, 5 square	15 g	11.0

Sliced Breads – Thin sliced pumpernickel (8.2 g/slice) is lowest and Sourdough (34.6 g/slice) is generally the highest.

Tortillas and Wraps – There are many low carb products on the market but be careful as some labels may be less than honest in their nutrition labels. Factory-made low carb wraps range between 3.0-19.0 grams net carbs. See the recipe in our Breads section and make your own.

Carb-Creeping Condiments

Bacon Bits, Imitation	1/2 oz	2.6
Cayenne Pepper, roasted, canned	1 ea	5.0
Garlic, minced, jarred	1 T	2.6
Horseradish, prepared	1 t	0.4
Mustard, Varied	1 t	0.1-1.0
Pickle, Dill, whole	4"	2.0
Pickle Relish	1T	3.3
Pickle, sweet	1 midget	1.2
Soy Sauce	1 T	1.2
Vinegar, Balsamic	1 T	2.7
Vinegar, Champagne	1 T	1.0
Vinegar, Cider	1 T	0.0
Vinegar, Red Wine	1 T	0.0
Vinegar, White	1 T	0.0
Vinegar, White Wine	1 T	1.5
Worcestershire Sauce	1 t	1.0

Cereals

Take a walk down the cereal aisle one day and check out the nutrition labels. A shame that foods we have thought to be healthful are actually loaded with carbohydrates, fillers and sugar.

Here are a few examples:

Alpen Muesli, No Sugar Added	1 cup	45.5 g
Cascadian Farm Organic Ancient Grains	1 cup	36g
Instant Cream of Wheat (original)	1.5 oz	32 g
Puffed Wheat	1 cup	10g
Rolled Oats (dry)	1/3 cup	19g
Special K	1 cup	21 g

Cheese

Many cheese products are prepared foods, always check the labels.

American	1 slice	1.5
Asiago	1 oz	0.5
Blue Cheese, Roquefort	1 oz	0.6
Brie	1 oz	0.1
Camembert	1 oz	0.1
Cheddar	1 oz	0.4
Cheez Whiz	2 T	5.6
Colby	1 oz	0.7
Cottage Cheese Curds, 2% fat	1 cup	8.2
Cream Cheese	1 T	1.0
Cream Cheese, Whipped	1 T	0.4
Edam	1 oz	0.4
Emmentaler	1 oz	0.0
Feta	1 oz	1.2
Goat, soft (Chèvre)	1 oz	0.3
Gouda	1 oz	0.6
Gruyère	1 oz	0.1
Havarti	1 oz	0.0
Jarlsberg	1 oz	1.2
Laughing Cow	1 wedge	1.0
Limburger	1 oz	0.1
Mascarpone	1 oz	0.0
Monterey Jack	1 oz	0.2
Mozzarella, fresh, balls	1 oz	0.0
Mozzarella, whole milk	1 oz	0.6
Parmesan, grated	1 T	0.2
Parmigiano-Reggiano, grated	1 T	0.0
Provolone	1 oz	0.6
Ricotta, Whole Milk	1 cup	7.6
Romano, grated	1 T	0.0
Swiss	1 oz	1.5
Velveeta	1 oz	2.8

Dairy & Dairy Substitutes

Butter	1 cup	0.1
Butter	1 T	0.0
Buttermilk	1 cup	11.7
Coffee-mate, powder	1t	1.0
Coffee Mate, Sugar-Free Vanilla, liquid	1 T	2.0
Coffee Mate, Hazelnut, liquid	1T	5.0
Cream, Half and Half	1 cup	10.4
Cream, Half and Half	1 T	0.3
Cream, Heavy	1 cup	6.6
Cream, heavy	1 T	0.4
Cream, Light	1 cup	7.1
Cream, Light	1 T	0.6
Ghee	1 t	0.0
Milk, 2 % milk	1 cup	12.0
Milk, Evaporated	1 cup	29.0
Milk, Goat's	1 cup	11.0
Milk, Skim	1 cup	12.0
Milk, Whole	1 cup	13.0
Sour Cream, regular	1 T	0.5
Sour Cream light	1 T	1.0
Sour Cream, non-fat	1 T	4.0
Yogurt, Greek Nonfat Plain	1 cup	9.0
Yogurt, Green Nonfat Flavored	6 oz	20.0
Yogurt, plain	1 cup	10.5-17.0
Yogurt, flavored	1 cup	30.0-50.0

Eggs

Raw, whole	1 egg	0.4
Raw, White only	1 ea	0.2
Dried Egg Whites	2 T	0.6
Egg Replacements	1 cup	1.6-8.0

Fish / Shellfish

Clams, Canned, drained	2 oz	3.3
Clams, Fresh, cooked	4 oz	5.8
Crab meat, canned or fresh	6 oz	0.0

Crab meat, Imitation	4 oz	7.0-15.0
Crab, Soft Shell, fried	1 med	10.5
Crawfish	6 oz	0.0
Fresh Fish	6 oz	0.0
Lobster, steamed	6 oz	1.5
Mussels, smoked, canned in oil	2 oz	2.5
Mussels, cooked	4 oz	8.4
Oysters, Eastern, Shelled	3 oz	2.3
Oysters, Pacific, Shelled	3 oz	4.2
Scallops	3 oz	2.7
Shrimp/Prawns, raw	3 oz	1.0
Squid, broiled	6 oz	6.4

Flours & Baking Supplies

Almond Flour	1 cup	12.0
Baking Soda	1/2 t	0.0
Baking Chocolate, Unsweetened	1 oz	4.1
Baking Powder	1/2 t	0.0
Cornmeal, yellow	1 cup	85.0
Cream of Tartar	1 t	1.8
Flaxseed, Ground	1 cup	0.0
Oat Flour	1 cup	48.4
Rice Flour, White	1 cup	120.0
Rye Flour, Medium	1 cup	64.8
Soy Flour	1 cup	21.6
Flour, White	1 cup	92.0
Flour, Whole Wheat	1 cup	73.0

Fruits

Apple, sliced	1/2 cup	6.4
Applesauce, unsweetened	1/2 cup	12.4
Apricot, sliced	1/2 cup	7.6
Banana, sliced	1/2 cup	15.2
Blackberries	1/2 cup	3.3
Blueberries	1/2 cup	9.0
Blueberries, frozen	1/2 cup	7.3
Boysenberries	1/2 cup	5.3
Cantaloupe, diced	1/2 cup	5.9

Cherries	1/2 cup	10.7
Clementine	1/2 cup	7.3
Coconut, Shredded Unsweetened	1/2 cup	2.5
Cranberries	1/2 cup	3.8
Dates, dried	1/2 cup	58.0
Figs, dried	1/2 cup	40.3
Gooseberries	1/2 cup	7.8
Grapefruit	1/2 cup	8.0
Grapes, Green Seedless	1/2 cup	13.0
Grapes, Purple Concord	1/2 cup	7.5
Grapes, Red Seedless	1/2 cup	13.0
Honeydew, diced	1/2 cup	7.3
Kiwi Fruit, sliced	1/2 cup	10.5
Mango	1/2 cup	11
Nectarine, sliced	1/2 cup	6.4
Orange	1/2 cup	8.5
Papaya	1/2 cup	6.6
Passionfruit	1/2 cup	15.4
Peaches, sliced	1/2 cup	6.5
Pear, Bartlett, sliced	1/2 cup	8.8
Pear, Asian, sliced	1/2 cup	4.3
Pineapple, sliced	1/2 cup	9.8
Plantains, sliced	1/2 cup	21.9
Raspberries	1/2 cup	3.1
Rhubarb	1/2 cup	1.7
Strawberries	1/2 cup	4.7

Grains

Barley, hulled, dry	1 cup	103.2
Quinoa, cooked	1 cup	34.4
Rice, brown, cooked	1 cup	84.8
Rice, white, cooked	1 cup	43.8
Rice, wild, cooked	1 cup	32.0
Whole Wheat, dry	1 cup	124.0

Herbs, Spices, Enhancers, Garnish

Most herbs and spices contain no carbs or miniscule amounts but watch out for spice mixtures spiked with sugar.

Allspice, ground	1 t	1.0
Anchovy Paste	1 T	0.0
Bacon Bits, real, jarred	1 oz	0.0
Bacon Bits, imitation	1 oz	1.6
Basil, fresh, chopped	1 T	0.0
Basil, dried	1 T	0.2
Bay Leaves, dried	1 ea	0.1
Capers, drained	1 T	0.2
Celery Salt	1 t	0.0
Jalapeño, fresh, sliced	1 cup	3.4
Chile Powder	1 T	0.0
Chives, dehydrated or fresh	1 T	0.1
Cilantro, fresh, chopped	1 T	0.0
Cinnamon, ground	1 t	0.7
Cloves, ground	1 t	0.6
Cocoa Powder, Unsweetened	1 T	1.3
Coriander, ground	1 t	0.0
Cumin Seed, ground	1 t	0.1
Curry Powder	1 T	0.0
Dill Weed, dried	1 T	1.3
Dill Weed, fresh, chopped	1 T	0.0
Garlic Minced, fresh or jarred	1 T	2.6
Garlic Powder	1 t	1.6
Garlic Salt	1 T	0.0
Ginger, ground	1 T	3.1
Ginger Root, fresh, grated	1 T	1.0
Lemon Zest, fresh, grated	1 T	0.3
Liquid Smoke	1 T	0.0
Mustard, Dijon	1 t	1.0
Mustard, Powder	1 t	0.4
Mustard, Yellow	1 t	0.1
Nutmeg, ground	1 t	0.6
Onion, minced, dried	1 T	3.7
Onion, powder	1 T	5.0
Orange Zest, fresh, grated	1 t	0.8
Oregano, dried	1 T	0.8
Paprika	1 T	1.3
Parsley, fresh, chopped	1 T	0.1
Pepper, black, ground	1 t	0.9

Pepper, red, crushed	1 t	0.5
Rosemary, dried	1 T	0.8
Sage, ground	1 t	0.1
Salt	1 t	0.0
Thyme, dried	1 T	0.8
Vanilla Extract	1 t	0.0

Nuts, Seeds, Legumes

Almonds	1 oz	2.3
Brazil nuts	1 oz	1.2
Cashews	1 oz	7.6
Chia Seeds	1 oz	1.0
Hazelnuts	1 oz	1.2
Macadamia nuts	1 oz	1.5
Pecans	1 oz	1.2
Peanuts	1 oz	2.1
Peanut Butter, smooth, commercial	1 oz	5.0
Pistachio nuts	1 oz	5.0
Pumpkin seeds	1 oz	3.9
Sunflower seeds	1 oz	2.3
Walnuts	1 oz	2.0

Meats

Muscle cuts and ground products from beef, lamb, pork, or poultry are carb-free except organ meats. Meats that have been altered (baked, cured, blended, corned, etc.) by a butcher or grocer will have their own (various) counts dependent upon the recipe or process.

Corned Beef	6 oz	0.8
Heart, Beef	4 oz	0.2
Liver, Beef	3.5 oz	3.9
Liver, Chicken	3.5 oz	0.7
Liver, Duck	3.5 oz	3.5
Tongue, Beef	3.5 oz	3.7

Meats, Prepared (approximations – always check labels)

Bacon, sliced (about 3 slices)	1 oz/28 g	0.2
Bologna	1 oz	2.0
Bratwurst	1 link	2.4
Canadian Bacon	2 slices	1.0
Chorizo	2 oz	1.1
Ham, Baked	1 oz	1.0
Ham, Honey Cured	1 oz	2.0
Kielbasa	2 oz	2.2
Knockwurst	1 link	2.3
Liverwurst	1 oz	1.0
Salami, Dry Cured	1 oz	0.5
Pastrami, Beef	4 oz	0.0
Pepperoni	6 oz	0.0
Prosciutto	6 oz	0.0
Roast Beef, Sliced	1 oz	0.6
Sausage, Italian Hot	2 oz	0.7
Sausage, Italian Sweet	2 oz	1.2
Turkey Sausage, Link (about 2)	2 oz/56 g	1.0

Sugar

Sugar, brown	1 t	4.0
Sugar, Brown, packed	1 cup	216.0
Sugar, white	1 t	4.0
Sugar, White	1 cup	200.0

Vegetables

Artichoke Hearts, marinated	1 cup	10.6
Artichoke Hearts, steamed	1 cup	15.7
Arugula	1 cup	0.4
Asparagus, 10 spears	1 cup	3.8
Avocado, Florida	1 cup	5.5
Avocado, Californian	1 cup	4.3
Bamboo Shoots, sliced, canned	1 cup	4.6
Beans, Green, steamed	1 cup	5.8
Beans, Yellow Wax, raw	1 cup	2.6
Beet Greens, steamed	1 cup	3.6

Beets, steamed, sliced	1 cup	13.6
Bok Choy, Steamed	1 cup	0.8
Broccoli, steamed	1 cup	3.6
Broccoli Raab (Rapini), steamed	1 cup	0.1
Brussels Sprouts, steamed	1 cup	4.3
Cabbage, Green/White, raw, shredded	1 cup	2.3
Cabbage, Savoy, raw, shredded	1 cup	2.1
Carrots, raw, shredded	1 cup	7.4
Cauliflower Florets, raw	1 cup	2.9
Celery, 1 stalk	8"	0.6
Chayote, steamed	1 cup	3.8
Corn, kernels, fresh	1 cup	25.2
Cucumber, raw, sliced	1 cup	3.2
Garlic, Minced	1 cup	42.1
Garlic, Minced	1 tsp	0.8
Jalapeño, fresh, sliced	1 cup	3.5
Lettuce, Boston or Bibb	1 cup	1.2
Lettuce, Iceberg	1 cup	1.3
Lettuce, Mesclun Mix	1 cup	2.0
Lettuce, Romaine	1 cup	0.6
Mushrooms, Button, sliced	1 cup	1.6
Mushrooms, Portobello, cooked	1 cup	1.6
Olives, Black	2 medium	0.9
Onion, cooked, chopped	1 cup	12.9
Onion, Red	1 cup	10.0
Onion, White	1 cup	14.0
Onion, Scallions	1 cup	4.0
Peas, fresh, shelled	1 cup	13.6
Peppers, Bell, Green	1 cup	4.4
Peppers, Bell, Red	1 cup	6.0
Potato, mashed	1 cup	32.1
Sauerkraut, drained	1 cup	2.4
Spaghetti Squash, baked	1 cup	8.0
Spinach	1 cup	1.0
Squash, Butternut, baked	1 cup	15.0
Squash, Hubbard, steamed	1 cup	8.4
Squash (summer), Yellow	1 cup	2.6
Squash (summer), Zucchini	1 cup	2.8
Sweet Potato, steamed, mashed	1 cup	34.8

Tomato, Cherry	1 cup	4.0
Tomato, Plum or Roma	1 cup	4.0
Tomato, Slicing	1 cup	5.0
Tomato Paste, canned	1 cup	39.0
Tomato Sauce, canned	1 cup	12.0-24.0
Tomato, stewed, canned	1 cup	13.2

CHAPTER 13

Vitamins & Supplements

We strongly suggest you take a multi-vitamin that is formulated specifically for your gender, exercise level, and age. Based on the structure and foods of this diet please ensure that your multi-vitamin contains potassium citrate (helps reduce the possibility of kidney stones), as well as ample magnesium.

Symptom Based Supplementation

You're not going to be as hungry as you were before you started this diet; therefore you'll be eating less. Eating less could result in a deficit of vital micro-nutrients. Your body will signal a deficit to you will illness or afflictions. To balance, correct, or heal the symptoms you might consider pill-based supplementation or foods that naturally supply the micro-nutrient.

This list is neither extensive nor presented as medical advice.

Vitamin A: acne, diarrhea, keratosis pilaris (bumps on upper arms), night blindness, infections (inner ear, respiratory system, urinary tract, vagina). Natural food sources: butter, cheese, cream, leafy vegetables, egg yolks, kidneys, liver.

Vitamin B2: anxiety, constipation, fatigue, headaches, irritability, muscle pain.
Natural food sources: kidneys, liver, pork.

Vitamin B3: abdominal pains, halitosis (bad breath), insomnia, irritability, fatigue, ulcers of the mouth.

Natural food sources: beef, chicken, fish, liver; smaller amounts in asparagus, leafy greens, mushrooms.

Vitamin B4: acne, anemia, dermatitis, dry lips, hair loss, itchy eyes.
Natural food sources: cream, eggs, leafy greens, oily fish, red meat.

Vitamin B6: confusion, depression, dermatitis, irritability, kidney stones.
Natural food sources: avocado, chicken, fish, nuts and seeds, red meat.

Vitamin B9: depression, diarrhea, forgetfulness, infertility.
Natural food sources: avocado, leafy greens and vegetables, liver, oranges.

Vitamin B12: agitation, depression, digestive trouble, constipation, moodiness, numbness in hands and feet, poor memory.
Natural food sources: dairy products, egg yolks, fish, red meat, shellfish.

Vitamin C: bleeding gums, dry scaly skin, fatigue, infections, joint pain, spider veins, muscle weakness, nose bleeds, wounds are slow to heal.
Natural food sources: citrus, green vegetables, peppers, tomatoes, berries.

Vitamin D: bone fractures, constipation, pelvic pain, lower back pain.
Natural food sources: eggs, fish liver oil, oily fish.

Vitamin E: impaired vision, infertility, loss of co-ordination.
Natural food sources: avocado, broccoli, leafy greens, peaches.

Calcium: brittle nails, eye twitches, muscle cramps, muscle twitches, weak bones.
Natural food sources: almonds, bok choy, broccoli, dairy products, kale, tofu, sesame seeds, watercress.

Chromium: fatigue, high cholesterol, glucose intolerance, increase in thirst, increase in urination.
Natural food sources: beef, cheese, egg yolks, nuts and seeds, oysters, poultry.

Coenzyme Q10: fatigue, frequent colds, irritability.
Natural food sources: fish, liver, meat.

Choline: decreased liver function, gallstones, high cholesterol.
Natural food sources: cauliflower, egg yolks, liver, meat, mushrooms, nuts and seeds.

Copper: depression, high blood pressure, insomnia, loss of hair and skin pigmentation, increased cholesterol.
Natural food sources: leafy greens, nuts and seeds, shellfish.

Iodine: chills, constipation, dry skin, fatigue, hair loss, menstrual irregularities, poor circulation, puffy face, weak muscles.
Natural food sources: fish, seafood, seaweed, iodized table salt.

Inosital: high cholesterol, intestinal trouble.
Natural food sources: seeds, wheat germ.

Iron: dizziness, fatigue, headaches, lack of motivation, restless leg syndrome, memory loss.
Natural food sources: asparagus, broccoli, fish, kale, liver, red meat, nuts and seeds, poultry, spinach.

Omega 3: acne, ADHD, blurred sight, dandruff, dry skin, slow healing of wounds.
Natural food sources: anchovies, flaxseed oil, halibut, hemp seeds oil, salmon, sardines, trout, tuna.

Magnesium: abdominal cramps, heart palpitations, irritability, menstrual cramps, muscle cramps, muscle twitches and spasms, vertigo.
Natural food sources: leafy greens, nuts, seafood.

Potassium: fatigue, irritability, insomnia, palpitations, poor concentration, weak muscles.
Natural food sources: apricots, bananas, figs, nuts and seeds, peaches, prunes.

Selenium: cataracts, infertility, lowered immune, muscle pain.
Natural food sources: brazil nuts, broccoli, dairy products, fish,

mushrooms, shellfish.

Silicon: bone fractures, gout.
Natural food sources: apples, avocado, citrus fruit, cucumber, garlic, guar gum, kelp, onion, strawberries.

Sodium: abdominal cramping, low blood pressure, poor circulation.
Natural food sources: dairy, eggs, meats, olives, soy sauce, spinach, watercress.

Zinc: acne, dandruff, dry skin, hair loss, infections, infertility, menstrual irregularities, slow wound healing, white spots under finger nails, low libido.
Natural food sources: brazil nuts, eggs, dairy, ginger root, liver, oysters, epitas, pecans, red meat.

Understanding Dopamine

When humans eat a big meal, our brains release dopamine.

Dopamine is a neurotransmitter that operates much like a 'feel good-- here's a reward' program. We eat, dopamine is released, and we catch a little buzz.

Through repetitive overeating we damage our natural dopamine activity. This damage is cumulative and worsens with repetitive insult.

Eventually our brain's satiety receptors, (the part of the brain responsible for telling us "You're full. Stop eating."), cease to function. Satiety receptors aren't affected as much by a full stomach as they are by the brain's knowing the food within the stomach contains the nutrients required to keep us alive and healthy. We are therefore capable of eating large quantities of food, our brain never telling us that we are satisfied, and no dopamine activity.

We eat, we're not nutritionally fed, and no buzz. Every day we repeat the process. As an example, consider the meal of a small fried chicken sandwich on a white bun. Theoretically that sandwich fills our tummy, satisfies our hunger, and at 12 ounces wouldn't be considered overeating. But that white bread, fried food, sugar, and all things processed confuse the brain's receptors. Our stomachs say "full" but our brains know that the food within is devoid of nutrients.

This damage to our receptors does not happen overnight, nor can it be repaired overnight. We have to give our brain some time to work this out and we can support the process with supplements.

Now that you know this you can now see how the early stages of switching to a nutrient dense and life-giving diet like KetoHybrid can be difficult.

You may know that you're feeding your body what it needs, but your dopamine receptors are still damaged, still clamoring for more because they're used to all that fast-burning processed stuff.

L-tyrosine

Enter tyrosine to save the day. Tyrosine is a natural supporter of dopamine. It is found in some foods you are or will be eating – chicken, duck, seaweed, ricotta cheese, wheat germ and dark chocolate.

The supplement version of tyrosine is L-tyrosine. It is an amino acid which aids in the process that repairs and reactivates healthy dopamine levels. This is not a quick fix to combat years of abuse. I took L-tyrosine supplements for a full month before I began eating KetoHybrid and felt that I needed to continue taking the supplement for two months after that.

Recommended dosage (by manufacturers and medical practitioners) for the average person is 500 to 1000 mg, twice daily, on an empty stomach.

DHA Omega 3

The next supporting supplement in the process is DHA Omega 3s. This supplement boosts dopamine levels by reducing production of the enzyme that breaks down dopamine.

DHA Omega 3 does more than that though. DHA is known for speeding up the receptors in the brain.

DHA Omega 3s are found naturally in salmon, tuna, and fish roe – all items on the KetoHybrid diet.

Recommended dosage for the average person is 600 to 1000 mg daily. You can also take a fish, algae or krill oil supplement to meet these levels, just be sure it is organic.

Finding The Best Supplements

Supplements and vitamins are available anywhere and everywhere. Like foodstuffs, this is a big, corporate-run, and corrupt industry. Companies change hands and corporations switch their formulations far too often. Purchase the wrong brand and you could just be throwing money down the toilet.

We will try to keep an eye on the better brands for you on the website[12] and welcome you to share your knowledge as well. Your owner-run, local health food store is also a safe bet for industry news and recommendations.

---

12 www.KetoHybrid.com/supplements

CHAPTER 14

Intro To Intermittent Fasting

As a natural progression in healthier nutrition you may want to add intermittent fasting to your regime. This is more than appropriate as KetoHybrid follows human genetic predisposition (the lifestyle of the caveman).

Fasting is a natural part of life and can happen quite accidentally.

Each of us experienced accidental fasting around our third month. We were so caught up in our day that we realized dinner time had passed us by and we hadn't eaten all day! Never would you have been able to convince either of us that this could happen. We just love our food too much!

We suggest that you also allow it to happen naturally. Your body knows how to speak to your brain. If it is hungry, tired, satiated, dehydrated, it passes along those messages. In the same sense, if it is not hungry (in the situation where it is quite content to burn up existing fat cells) you won't be signaled to eat.

On the days that we weren't signaled, nearly 24 hours had passed. Neither one of us were performing strenuous tasks on those days. This may have been why our bodies were content to hum along on stored fat. On the days leading up to our individual fasts we did notice that we had been less hungry at every meal.

You could force a fast if you are interested in trying it. Keep it short and listen to your body. If your body starts screaming for food, by all means end the fast early and try again on another day.

A short fast:

- Forces your body to burn up more stored fat.
- Makes you feel lighter and more energetic.
- May reduce glucose levels, blood pressure, and cholesterol.
- More toxins are released.
- A measurable increase in HGH (human growth hormone) based on scientific trials.
- A metabolic reset, followed by an increase in metabolic rate.
- An increase in good gut bacteria.

You won't want to take your fast past the two-day mark as your metabolism will slow down and your body may believe that it needs to hold back on the fat cells as starvation is imminent. At that point cortisol production will increase, amino acids will be released and muscle tissue will begin deteriorating. You'll notice it all through weariness and exhaustion.

Easy Intermittent Fasting

The easiest way to try a short fast is on the back on a good night's sleep. Sleeping is still fasting so if you want to try an 18 hour fast, plan on having your last meal four hours before bed, sleep a full eight hours, and don't take your first meal until you've been awake for six hours.

Techniques for intermittent fasting are as individual as you are. If you try it and enjoy the way it makes you feel, let us know. We'll be researching and experimenting more on this topic soon.

Be sure, as always, to continue drinking ample water during a fast to flush out toxins.

CHAPTER 15

Organic or Not?

Even though we would prefer a fully organic diet, our household budgets don't always allow for this. Choosing organic foods will add years to your life. Speculatively, choosing heirloom foods (non-GMO), will add even more.

Some foods that are more susceptible to chemical use and some more resilient. The EWG (Environmental Working Group) regularly tests the American food supply and publishes a list of the best and worst cases of pesticide and chemical contamination. The sample below is directly from their website5 at the time of writing.

Must Buy Organic:
- All meats
- Eggs
- Berries and cherries
- Broccoli
- Bananas, apples and pears
- Cauliflower
- Tomatoes and peppers
- Spinach, lettuce or any other leafy green
- Peaches, nectarines or any other stone fruit
- Grapes
- Celery
- Green Onions
- Cucumbers
- Oranges and Tangerines
- Honeydew Melon

- Zucchini
- Carrots
- Green Beans
- Any food item you eat a lot of. The chemical residues that are causing us harm are cumulative. So even if your favorite food isn't on this list, if you eat it often, you need to add "only organic" to your list.

Less Likely to Be Tainted (be sure to wash well anyway)
- Coconut
- Onions
- Avocado
- Honey
- Asparagus
- Sweet Potato
- Oysters, clams, and mussels
- Eggplant
- Grapefruit
- Kiwi
- Mangos
- Mushrooms
- Papaya
- Pineapples
- Cabbage
- Cantaloupe

CHAPTER 16

Meals, Meal Plans, and More

KetoHybrid aims to spark an interest in nutrition, connect you to your satiety level, understand your emotional ties with food, and to recognize food addictions, if any.

We believe meal plans hinder those aims and stymie creativity. It is important that you love your meals.

Equally important that you are able to make sound decisions when life serves up a hectic schedule. You can grill up some meat and vegetable as quickly as hitting a fast food window. Make a stir fry faster than waiting on a pizza delivery. With a little forethought and freezer space – you can also make multiple meals at a time instead of just one.

This is empowerment, not dictation. Not one of us needs to be controlled any more than we already are by family, time constraints, financial obligations, employment, and government. You are in charge of and responsible for, what you eat and how much you eat.

With that said, we do understand that this may be a new way of eating for you. Counting net carbs or 'looking after macros' could be a major disruption in consumption habits. Without a clear view snacks and meals are hard to envision. "What's left to eat without bread? Without pasta? Without rice?"

We were there not long ago. We had read the rules and understood the concepts behind low carb, Paleo-influenced, and Ketogenic diets. Translating those rules to our daily diet took more than a few weeks.

We were scared of being hungry or feeling deprived. We fretted over increasing fat intake. We decided that our weight couldn't get much worse and jumped in, in spite of our fears. We made mistakes, conferred a lot, and corrected our intake. It was laborious but all worth it; especially so now that we have committed ourselves to helping others.

Neither Veronica nor I (aged 20 and 50 respectively with two very different levels of activity) have counted calories. As you may have seen on social and national news networks, Veronica lost the majority of her weight in the first 10 weeks. From a plus size dress to her high school jeans in 2 1/2 months.

In the beginning we put our trust in the high fat ideal and poured on the butter and cream. We ate blocks of cheese like they were going out of style. A pound of bacon could disappear between us in a few days – just as snacks. While she was at work all day, I popped almonds at my desk and noshed on fatty salami.

Veronica is now a few pounds from her goal weight and will simply continue to eat the way we have learned. As I write this last section of the book I'm still 15 pounds away from my goal. I blame my test kitchen for my slow progress but in reality I have been known to cheat and set myself back by many days.

When we charted our progress and checked in with other dieters, it became more important to get this information in as many hands as possible, as soon as possible, than losing the last pounds.

I've learned my lesson about cheating and am more committed than ever. I'm out of the test kitchen and nearly finished the long hours of writing and lack of sleep that went with it. This book is in the final stages of completion (end of May 2014). I fully and realistically expect to be at my goal weight within the next six weeks. I'll make a final progress report[13], if you'd like to check in on me.

What follows are a few meals you might find on your plate; plus 5 typical days that are low in net carbs, have relatively balanced macros, and equate to less than 1900 calories per day.

That is our suggested order of priority.

---

13 http://www.KetoHybrid.com/progress-laura

Priority 1: Low Net Carbs
Priority 2: Balanced Macros
Priority 3: Calories

Eat your meals slowly and tune into your body. Wait ten to 15 minutes before you take a second helping. Don't worry about much else unless you hit a plateau. Only at that time should you drive yourself crazy counting every calorie that passes your lips.

We invite you to skip a meal if you aren't hungry, to leave food on your plate when you're satiated, to snack on safe foods if you are hungry, to increase portion sizes (with macro balance and within reason), and let your body take care of putting the food or fat-burning processes to efficient use.

Daily Considerations

- A good multivitamin, taken with food that contains fat
- Broth, 2 cups (supplements sodium and other nutrients that you aren't getting on this diet, cuts cravings, prevents diet fatigue)
- Vegetables, at least 2 cups per day (this will/should eat up your daily carb allowance). We chose broccoli, zucchini, spinach, cauliflower, and mushrooms as our go to staples. You can choose any other low-carb leafy green or fibrous vegetable (see list in next chapter).

Sample Plates

Very basic and quick meals including net carbs, calories and (somewhat) balanced macros. Pick and choose, find your own favorites in the recipe section, and alter any ingredients with the help of the net carb counter in the previous chapter.

Your nutrition and your health are your responsibility and you're going to do a great job of it from this point forward!

Tuna Salad Sandwiches (Lettuce Wraps)
1/2 can tuna (packed in water, 3.1 ounces) mixed with 2 tbsp homemade mayonnaise and 1 chopped green onion, 4 ounces lettuce leaves (3-4 large, wrapped around the tuna salad)
371 calories; F 71 P 26 C 3; net carb 1.4

Scrambled Eggs with Spinach & Bacon
2 eggs, 1/2 cup spinach, 1 slice bacon (cooked and chopped), 1/2 tsp salt; cooked in 1 tbsp butter
315 calories; F 70 P 24 C 6; net carb 1.9

Pork Chop with Mac and Cheese
1 pork chop 3/4" thick, with 1 serving of Faux Mac & Cheese
489 calories; F 60 P 37 C 3; net carb 4.0

Guacamole with Dippers
1 avocado mashed with 1 tbsp olive oil, 1/2 tsp minced garlic, 1/2 tsp sea salt, 1 tbsp lemon juice
plus 10 Big Dippers (recipe from this book)
calories 429; F 82 P 3 C 14; net carb 4.9

Chicken Wings
4 chicken wings rolled in 1/4 cup of Parmesan and 1 tsp garlic, baked
1 cup cauliflower
4 pieces of celery (approximately 4") with 1 ounce blue cheese dip
690 calories; F 61 P 33 C 6; net carb 6.1

Burrito
1/4 pound ground beef, 2 ounces shredded cheddar cheese, 1 ounce sour cream, 1 cup lettuce leaves, 1/4 cup diced tomato, 1 flax seed wrap, 1/4 cup diced red onion
609 calories; F 68 P 26 C 6; net carb 6.2

Tuna Salad Plate
1/2 can tuna (packed in water, 3.1 ounces) mixed with 2 tbsp homemade mayonnaise and 1 chopped green onion, 2 ounces lettuce leaves (about 3 large), 2 hard boiled eggs, 1/4 tsp sea salt, juice of 1/2 lemon
551 calories; F 67 P 28 C 4; net carb 6.3

Asparagus Swiss Omelet
omelet: 1/2 cup cooked asparagus, 2 eggs, 1 ounce swiss cheese, 2 tbsp heavy cream
side: 1/2 cup cauliflower, 3 tbsp hollandaise
396 calories; F 69 P 24 C 7; net carb 6.3

Soy Sauce Chicken

4 ounces of chicken breast cut into strips and cooked in 2 tbsp sesame oil; topped with soy sauce (a mix of 2 ounces soy sauce, 1/2 tsp minced garlic, 1/4 tsp ground ginger)
3/4 cup shredded cabbage with 2 ounces of sliced mushrooms braised in 1 tbsp butter
522 calories; F 71 P 22 C 7; net carb 6.7

BLT: Bacon, Lettuce, and Tomato

4 slices bacon, 1 large slice tomato, 1 large lettuce leaf, 1 ounce mayonnaise, KetoHybrid bun or 2 small slices of KetoHybrid whole wheat bread (from this book)
302 calories; F 70 P 17 C 13; net carb 7.6

Hamburger

4 ounces ground beef burger, 2 ounces cheddar, 1 tomato slice, 1 ounce mayonnaise, 1 large lettuce leaf
1 KetoHybrid burger bun
675 calories; F 72 P 22 C 6; net carb 7.9

Sirloin Steak

4 ounces sirloin
4 ounces mushrooms and 2 ounces onion sauteed in 1 ounce butter
1/4 pound asparagus spears
513 calories; F 71 P 21 C 8; net carb 8.6

Salmon Dinner

4 oz salmon grilled with 1/2 ounce olive oil, 2 cups steamed broccoli with 1 ounce grated cheddar cheese melted on top, 2 ounces mushrooms lightly sauteed in 1/2 ounce butter
514 calories; F 65 P 28 C 7; net carb 9.1

Warm Spinach Salad

3 cups fresh spinach topped with 2 ounces cheddar, chopped bacon (1 slice) and egg(1 hard boiled) with a warmed dressing (a mix of 1 ounce bacon fat, 1 ounce home made mayo, 1 tsp water and 1/2 tsp black pepper)
691 calories; F 74 P 19 C 6; net carb 10.3

Zucchini Noodles with Chicken
2 cups of zucchini noodles and 2 ounces of cooked chicken, drizzled with olive oil and fresh basil
376 calories; F 65 P 25 C 6; net carb 7.7

Snacks

We snack every day, multiple times per day. When traveling, jerky and nuts work well and will save you from the perils of a fast food checkout line. Bring your lunch to work but always throw in a little extra – sliced meat, cheese, hard boiled egg – in case you get hungry.

Snacks with (nearly) Reckless Abandon:

- bone broth (chicken or beef)
- home made beef jerky
- 1-2 slices home made bacon
- hard boiled egg
- 1-2 slices deli meat (no additives, no more than 1 gram carbohydrate per serving)
- deli meat slice wrapped around a cucumber spear
  a few pork rinds (homemade or find an additive-free source)
- a few cooked shrimp (cooked in butter, dipped in horseradish)

Sample Snack Ideas (in Moderation):

- 1 tablespoon of coconut oil (right out of the jar or frozen in 1 tbsp portions – honestly, this sounds disgusting but the research backs that this assists in weight loss6. It also immediately quiets hunger).
- 1/2 cup sauerkraut
- 1-2 ounces of hard cheese
- 1/2 avocado with sea salt, black pepper and a small squirt of lime or lemon
- 2-3 celery sticks with 1/2 ounce blue cheese dressing
- 1/2 cup fresh or frozen blackberries or raspberries
- 1/4 cup of brazil nuts, pecans, or pumpkin seeds

Sample Days

Note that in a few of these days there is ample 'wiggle' room for adding in your favorite foods and snacks, even if they contain carbs.

Day 1
1 egg, 2 slices bacon
1 cup spinach, 3 ounces cheddar cheese, 1 tbsp oil, few green pepper slices, salt/pepper
2 ounces salami
2 cups broth
4 ounces chicken, 2 cups asparagus, 1 ounce Hollandaise sauce, 1 tbsp olive oil, 2 tbsp Parmesan
2 keto cookies

Daily calories: 1543
F: 69, P: 24, C: 8
Net Carb: 13.5

Day 2
ketohybrid classic breakfast sandwich (#1)
3 ounces tuna, 1 green onion, 1 tbsp mayo, salt/pepper, 2 ounces cheddar cheese
2 cups broth
4 oz burger patty, 1 ounce Swiss cheese, 2 cups broccoli
ketohybrid bun with 1 ounce almond butter

excluding breakfast sandwich 550 cal and 3 net keto bun (146 cal 2.9 net)
1761 calories
F: 67 P: 26 C: 9
Net Carb: 20.9

Day 3
1/2 cup blackberries
3 ounces chicken breast on 1 cup spinach leaves, with 1 slice crumbled bacon, 1 tbsp mayo
2 ounces cheddar cheese
4 ounces pork roast
1 1/2 cup cauliflower with 3 tbsp Hollandaise sauce

1 cup broth

1133 calories
F: 62, P: 30, C: 7
Net Carb: 16.2

Day 4
coffee with double cream
keto breakfast sand #2
french onion soup with extra cup of broth
shephard's pie
1/2 keto mini chocolate cheesecake

1880 calories
F: 66, P: 19 C: 15
Net Carb: 19.6

Day 5
coffee with double cream
frittata
coffee with double cream
leafy Mediterranean salad
chicken schnitzel
1 cup broccoli
2 ounces almonds
1 tbsp coconut oil

1624 calories
F: 58, P: 22, C: 20
Net Carb: 24

Weekly Meal Plan – Veronica

Veronica recently moved closer to her job, in her own apartment and with only a small freezer. As a single dieter, this is her weekly food plan and her weekly shopping list.

We thought it might be of some use or interest to you in your own planning.

Monday
2 eggs with 1 cup spinach and 2 slices bacon
broth
Chicken & Spinach w/Bacon
Pork Chop with Faux Mac & Cheese

Tuesday
2 eggs with 2 slices bacon
broth
Chicken & Broccoli Salad, Caesar dressing
Warm Spinach Salad

Wednesday
Blackberries
broth
Chicken & Cheese Salad 3 ounces chicken breast, 2 ounces cheddar
cheese
Roast Pork with Cauliflower and Hollandaise

Thursday
Blackberries
Guacamole and Dippers
Salmon with Mac/Cheese

Friday
Scrambled Eggs with Spinach & Bacon
broth
Beef Burrito in Golden Flax Wrap
Steak & Asparagus

Saturday
3 Minute Blueberry Muffin
Caesar Salad
broth
Soy Sauce Chicken with Cabbage and Mushrooms

Sunday
Eggs Benedict
broth

Tuna Salad Wraps
Burger Patty with the Toppings
Cauliflower

Shopping List for Weekly Meal Plan – Veronica

12 eggs + 2 yolks
6 slices bacon
2 slices peameal
14 ounces chicken breast
1 pork chop 3/4" thick
4 ounce sirloin
8 ounces pork tenderloin
1/2 pound ground beef
4 ounce salmon steak
soup bones

large package spinach (5 1/2 cups projected)
small broccoli (1/2 - 1 cup projected)
romaine or iceberg lettuce (2.5 cups projected)
red onion (1/4 cup projected)
1 plum tomato (1/4 cup diced + 1 slice projected)
small bunch asparagus
2 small cauliflower (6.5 cups projected)
1 small cabbage (3/4 cup projected)
small package mushrooms (2 ounces projected)
1 green onion
garlic (3 cloves projected)
small package blackberries
small package raspberries
1 avocado
1 lemon

16 ounces cheddar cheese
1 ounce sour cream
3 ounces cream cheese
1 cup Parmesan cheese

Need on hand:
1/4 cup chia seeds
1/4 cup pepitas (pumpkin seeds)
1/4 cup sunflower seeds
1/4 cup sesame seeds, raw
1 tbsp coconut flour
1 tbsp psyllium husks
1 1/4 cups golden flax seeds, ground

sesame oil
coconut oil
olive oil
butter
anchovy paste
soy sauce
dijon mustard
worcestershire sauce
white wine vinegar

sea salt
baking powder
baking soda
onion powder
garlic powder
vanilla extract

Sunday 'To Do' List for Weekly Menu Plan - Veronica

1. make broth
2. make mayo
3. make 1/2 full recipe for Caesar salad dressing (partial left)
4. make 1/2 full recipe for Hollandaise (partial left)
5. make faux mac and cheese (2 portions will be leftover for the following week)
6. make 1/2 recipe dippers (2 portions will be leftover for snacks or the following week)
7. make 1/2 golden flax wraps (1 large or 2 small wraps will be leftover)

8. cook pork tenderloin (1 portion will be leftover for snacks or for the following week)

Weekly Meal Plan - Laura

Working from home no more than 10 feet from the fridge door. No daily commute or demands on my time. Happy to spend a little extra time in the kitchen. Eating when hungry including snacks of homemade broth, meats, cheese, spinach salad and zucchini fritters.

Adapt any day to include intermittent fasting by moving menu choices around to suit your own schedule.

Saturday
Today's Focus: Grocery shopping – 1 hour plus travel time
Key notes: Your fridge is bare this morning, but you don't want to shop hungry.
Breakfast – If you still have 2 eggs, whip up a "Use-It-Up Frittata"! It's the same recipe as the Favorite Frittata but you toss in any cooked leftover vegetables or meats you have on hand that taste great together. Now go shopping before you get hungry again.
Lunch – Caesar salad
Dinner – Roast chicken and gravy (gravy can be thickened with chia seeds), faux mashed potatoes (made from cauliflower), green beans, and sauteed rapini.
Snack safely to satiation throughout the day. Stop eating after dinner.

Sunday
Today's Focus: Big Prep Day for the Week Ahead – 2.5 hours
Breakfast – Eggs Florentine in ramekins (so easy).
Lunch – Hamburger sliders with zucchini patties. (Cook twice the hamburger patties that you'll eat tonight. Make the full zucchini patty recipe – you'll eat them up later in the week.)
Dinner – Grilled tuna steak with asparagus. (Cook twice the tuna that you'll eat tonight, we'll use two half portions later in the week.)
Snack safely to satiation throughout the day. Stop eating after dinner.

Monday
Breakfast – Grab a 2 pack of muffins and eat them at your desk.
Lunch – Chicken salad, or soup made from broth (I made the broccoli

chowder during this week and include those ingredients in the shopping list below) with a few zucchini patties.

Dinner – 4 grilled shrimp on a warm spinach salad.

Snack safely to satiation throughout the day. Stop eating after dinner.

Tuesday

Breakfast – Fresh berries with almonds.

Lunch – Tuna salad with walnuts (using 1/2 of the extra tuna portion from Sunday)

Dinner – Asian Chicken and Broccoli (modified from the beef version in the recipes section and using leftover chicken from Saturday night's dinner)

Snack safely to satiation throughout the day. Stop eating after dinner.

Wednesday

Breakfast – 1 egg, 2 large shrimp, and spinach – scrambled.

Lunch – Hamburger patty (from Sunday's lunch prep) with aioli sauce and a vegetable.

Dinner – Salad Nicoise (using 1 of the hard boiled eggs and 1/2 of the extra tuna portion from Sunday night's prep)

Snack safely to satiation throughout the day. Stop eating after dinner.

Thursday

Morning Task: Get Ropa Vieja in the slow cooker on low, with a timer for 8 hours. Add 3/4 cup of water if you'll be gone for 9 hours.

Evening Task: Roast pork belly.

Breakfast – 2 muffins

Lunch – 1 hard boiled egg with fresh herbs and lettuce salad

Dinner - Ropa Vieja with roasted cauliflower (cook twice what you'll eat tonight).

Snack safely to satiation throughout the day. Stop eating after dinner.

Friday

Breakfast – A few strips of home made bacon with leftover roasted cauliflower. Cook an extra strip for your lunch salad.

Lunch – Green salad with bacon and any dressing (if you have leftover aioli whip it into any vinaigrette for a creamy dressing).

Dinner – Pork chops, faux mashed potatoes, vegetable.

Snack safely to satiation throughout the day. Stop eating after dinner.

Shopping List for Weekly Meal Plan - Laura

You will have leftovers to snack on, or eat later in the month. These include bacon, 8 muffins and 2 heat-and-eat broccoli soups in the freezer, a lunch meal of Ropa Vieja and your staples.

Romaine - enough for 1 salad
Boston Lettuce - enough for 1 large salad
Spinach - enough for 2 salads

Fresh herbs - thyme, basil, oregano,
3 small cauliflower (or 2 large)
3 whole broccoli
2 servings green veg of choice (your favorite or a seasonal item)
1 1/2 serving of green beans
3 zucchini
3 lb bag of onions
bunch of green onions
1 medium red onion
small bundle of asparagus
red bell pepper
2 hot peppers
thumb-sized piece of ginger

6-7 tomatoes
1 avocado
1 lemon
1 lime

pint strawberries
pint blueberries
pint raspberries

4 oz almonds
4 oz walnuts

12 eggs

1 whole chicken

1 pound hamburger
1 lb flank steak
2 pork chops
1 lb pork belly, skin on

6 large shrimp
2 tuna steaks

almond flour
tapioca flour

black olives
anchovy paste

Considerations:

- More almonds (or other nuts if you like them as a small snack)
- More berries or citrus fruit if you like to add some to your water

You'll need these, do you have enough?

snacking salami and cheese
heavy whipping cream (for coffee)

fresh garlic
horseradish

baking soda
baking powder (gluten-free)
unrefined sea salt

coconut oil
olive oil
vanilla extract
unrefined sea salt
white vinegar
balsamic vinegar
capers

Dried Spices: mustard, peppercorns, cumin, coriander, fennel seed, bay leaves, thyme, rosemary, mustard seeds, allspice, cinnamon, chili powder, oregano

Sunday 'To Do' List for Weekly Menu Plan - Laura

1. Half of last night's leftover chicken makes a chicken salad for a mid-week lunch. The other half is stored for Tuesday night's dinner.
2. Simmer bones into chicken broth or make a bone broth from purchased soup bones. Freeze half the broth for another week.
3. Grate zucchini for today's lunch recipe.
4. Boil 4 eggs and store in their shells, in the refrigerator.
5. Bake blueberry muffins and wrap in plastic, 2 to a package.
6. Make mayonnaise, set aside 1/2 for aioli.
7. Make a salad dressing for the week.
8. Cure pork belly for homemade bacon.

CHAPTER 17

Soups & Appetizers

Soup is magical. It slows down the speed eaters, can be packed with vital nutrition, is generally low in calories, and it fills you up so you're less likely to overeat.

Our busy lifestyles have all but killed the tradition of a soup starter. We don't have time to create a great broth, we buy boneless cuts of meat to save prep time of meals, and even when we do have bones we're quick to toss them in the trash.

Let me help you to put soup back on the menu!

Soup, stock, or broth – which is it?

While trained chefs may disagree, for the purpose of this book and nutritional counts, I distinguish them as such:

> **Soup** – a fully finished, on-the-table, food that is started with a stock or broth.
> **Stock** – usually a base for soup that, (other than water) contains multiple ingredients.
> **Broth** – a base for soup that is neither flavored, nor fortified, by any item other than the main ingredient.

I've always enhanced soup stock by adding ingredients during the first boiling down phase – namely carrots, onions, potatoes, and garlic. I had never considered that those carbs would stick around in my healthy broth after being boiled down and removed with bones, gristle and skin.

The USDA Nutrition Database confirms my worst fears; carb counts for homemade soups are high.

To illustrate this clearly, if we make the chicken soup recipe below using a homemade stock, net carbs per cup is 9+ grams. Made with a homemade broth, net carbs per cup is 2 grams.

The Nutrition Database's lowest carb soups are broth-based – specifically from dehydrated bouillon. Bouillon is available everywhere in dry cubes or liquid. You can also find ready-to-serve Certified Organic broth, prepared from bouillon. In a pinch for time or if you're out of homemade stock purchase an organic bouillon (trust that non-organic and overly processed meat and poultry products are not something you want in your body).

Getting Into The Swing of Soups

When you buy any cut of meat (poultry included) you'll pay less per pound if you remove it from the bone at home. You don't need to learn a new skill or be a perfectionist about the task – nothing goes to waste as whatever is left on the bone will be fortifying your future soup stock.

Dedicate an entire shelf in your freezer to soup-making. One bag for beef bones, one for chicken, and one for vegetables. Add to these throughout the month and when you either have time or ample amounts in a bag, make your stock or broth.

Buy marrow or soup bones from the butcher if you're not eating much beef off the bone. For less than $5 we purchase enough bones to make 4 gallons of beef stock, then divide it into equal portions of stock and broth.

Cream of Mushroom Soup

Yield: 6 servings
Serving Size: 1 cup
Net Carbs per Serving: 4.1 g
Prep Time: 5 minutes
Cook Time: 15-20 minutes

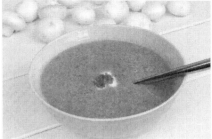

1 tbsp butter
2 tbsp onion, minced
1⁄4 tsp thyme, dried
4 cups mushrooms, coarsely chopped (1 pound)
1⁄2 bay leaf
1 tsp salt
1⁄2 tsp fresh-ground black pepper
4 cups chicken broth
1 cup half & half cream

1. Melt butter in a 6 cup stock pot and saute onions for 5 minutes or until translucent. Add mushrooms and spices and continue sauteing until the mushrooms are cooked (they're cooked when water begins to accumulate in the pan).
2. Carefully transfer mushroom and onions to a food processor and chop without pureeing completely.
3. Return mushrooms to the stock pot, add soup stock and simmer for 10 minutes more.
4. Add cream and simmer 2 minutes more.
5. Serve immediately.

Amount Per Serving	
Calories	106.94
Calories From Fat (72%)	77.45

Total Fat 8.73g	
Saturated Fat 4.8g	72%
Cholesterol 24.68mg	
Sodium 502.24mg	17%
Potassium 219.15mg	11%
Total Carbohydrates 4.72g	
Fiber 0.59g	
Sugar 1.8g	KetoHybrid
Protein 3.38g	2014

Mini Mock Matzo Ball Soup

Traditional Matzo Ball soup has been a favorite of ours for years, but we don't enjoy eating all those carbohydrates. The average one cup measure of traditionally made matzo ball soup hides 9.2 net carbs in that salty broth. Compare that to a cup of this recipe at only 2.2 net carbs – plus the macros have better balance.

We increased the portion size to 1 1/2 cups and still kept the net carbs at a respectable level. A perfect starter to a light dinner or as a lunch alternative.

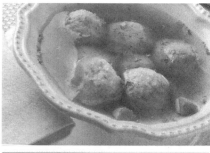

Yield: 4 servings

Net Carbs per Serving: 3.3 g

Serving Size: 1/4 recipe (about 1 1/2 cup stock plus 6 mini matzo balls)

Prep Time: 10 minutes

Cook Time: 20 minutes

Time to Table: 2+ hours

2 cups almond flour, blanched

4 eggs

1 tsp salt

1/2 tsp pepper

6 cups homemade chicken broth

1/3 cup carrots, cut into thin strips or small wedges

Amount Per Serving	
Calories	204.91
Calories From Fat (68%)	140.22

Total Fat 15.29g		
Saturated Fat 3.07g		68%
Cholesterol 196.5mg		
Sodium 873.24mg		
Potassium 124.41mg		23%
Total Carbohydrates 4.66g		9%
Fiber 1.32g		
Sugar 2.12g		KetoHybrid
Protein 10.89g		2014

1. Beat eggs with salt and pepper until frothy (about 2 minutes).
2. Stir in almond flour, mix well, and refrigerate for 2 hours to set.
3. In a medium sized pot, boil 6 cups of water with a teaspoon of salt.
4. Roll refrigerated mix into 24 small balls (1" in diameter) and add to the pot of boiling water.
5. Reduce heat and allow to simmer for 20 minutes.
6. In a separate pot, heat chicken stock to serving temperature.
7. Serve each bowl of stock with 6 matzo balls. Garnish with a pinch of chopped parsley or minced scallion.
8. If storing leftovers, continue to keep the mock matzo balls separate from the broth until use.

Chicken Soup

Made with homemade broth a soup serves up a healthy and satisfying meal. Some amazing soups are made the day before grocery shopping, when cooked meats and vegetable dishes need to be used up to make room in the refrigerator.

Now that you know the carb counts (if you don't, you can quickly reference many food items in this book) of meats and vegetables, you're sure to make good decisions of how much of each item to include per serving. I've included the ingredient list and nutritional data for a soup we eat most often.

Yield: 2 servings
Serving Size: 1/2 recipe, about 10 ounces
Net Carbs per Serving: 2.4 grams
Prep Time: 10 minutes
Cook Time: 30 minutes

2 cups chicken broth
1/4 cup cauliflower, cooked and chopped
1/2 cup chicken breast, cooked, diced, skinless
1/2 cup spinach leaves, raw and coarsely chopped
1/4 tsp red pepper flakes
1/2 tsp onion powder

1. Heat broth to a simmer in a medium saucepan.
2. Add chicken, spices and cauliflower to the stock.
3. Split spinach into two equal portions and place in serving bowl. Ladle soup over spinach and serve.

Amount Per Serving	
Calories	102.65
Calories From Fat (39%)	39.62

Total Fat 4.32g	
Saturated Fat 1.37g	
Cholesterol 36.75mg	
Sodium 179.01mg	
Potassium 189.74mg	
Total Carbohydrates 2.87g	
Fiber 0.51g	
Sugar 1.31g	
Protein 12.37g	

39%
11%
51%

KetoHybrid
2014

Creamy Chicken Chowder

The chicken soup above is wonderful but if your fat intake for the day is low, consider this chowder instead.

Yield: 3 servings
Serving Size: 1/3 recipe, about 9 ounces
Net Carbs per Serving: 2.8 grams
Prep Time: 10 minutes
Cook Time: 30 minutes

2 cups chicken broth
1/2 cup cauliflower, cooked and chopped
1/2 cup chicken breast, cooked, diced, skinless
1/2 tsp onion powder
1/2 cup heavy cream

1. Heat broth to a simmer in a medium saucepan.
2. Add chicken, spices and cauliflower to the stock and heat through (2-3 minutes).
3. Add cream right before serving and heat through (1-2 minutes).

Amount Per Serving	
Calories	206.21
Calories From Fat (75%)	155.53

Total Fat 17.56g	
Saturated Fat 10.05g	75%
Cholesterol 78.84mg	
Sodium 132.97mg	6%
Potassium 153.26mg	18%
Total Carbohydrates 3.25g	
Fiber 0.39g	
Sugar 1.06g	KetoHybrid
Protein 9.08g	2014

French Onion Soup

Worried you have to eat French onion soup naked forever more? Take heart! With any of the bread recipes in this book you can have your soup with cheese crouton and eat it too! I've calculated 1/2 of a slice (2 x 4") from the Low Carb Bagels and Bread recipe* per bowl of soup in the nutritional data below.

Yield: 4 servings
Serving Size: 1 1/4 cup of soup
plus bread/cheese topping
Net Carbs per Serving: 6.0 grams
Prep Time: 15-20 minutes
Cook Time : 45 minutes

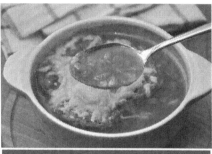

1 1/2 cups onions, yellow, thinly sliced

4 tbsp butter

4 cups homemade beef broth

1/4 tsp onion powder

2 slices of low carb bread, halved

2 tbsp butter

1/4 tsp garlic powder

4 slices Swiss cheese (one ounce per slice)

Amount Per Serving	
Calories	374.67
Calories From Fat (81%)	301.62
Total Fat 34.18g	
Saturated Fat 17.71g	
Cholesterol 78.88mg	
Sodium 253.83mg	
Potassium 89.12mg	
Total Carbohydrates 7.36g	
Fiber 1.39g	
Sugar 1.4g	
Protein 10.57g	

KetoHybrid
2014

1. In a medium size stock pot over medium high heat, saute onions in butter for 8-10 minutes or until slightly carmelized.
2. Turn down heat, add broth and onion powder. Simmer for 20-30 minutes.
3. Make soup croutons by lightly toasting 2 slices of low carb bread in 2 tablespoons of butter with garlic salt in a non-stick frying pan. Each serving of soup will have one crouton, approximately 2" x 4" in size.
4. Preheat oven to 375°F.
5. Put 4 ovenproof bowls onto a cookie sheet, and ladle hot soup into the bowls. Top each bowl with one crouton and a slice of swiss cheese and place into the oven for about 15 minutes or until the cheese has softly bubbled.
6. Serve immediately.

*Or any equivalent bread with a similar value of 0.7 net carbs, 2.7 grams fat, and 32 calories per bowl of soup.

Bean-Free Chili

This won't be a traditional chili, but it will give you the satisfaction of flavor. To keep net carbs low you'll want to use a red onion (also known as Bermuda) and fresh tomatoes. I'm suggesting a plum tomato (also known as Roma) as they have more flesh, less water, per ounce.

Yield: 4 servings
Serving Size: 1 cup
Net Carbs per Serving: 4.0 grams
Prep Time: 5 minutes
Cook Time: 50-60 minutes

1⁄4 cup red onion, chopped
1⁄4 cup green pepper, diced
1⁄4 cup mushrooms, sliced
1 pound ground beef
2 cups plum tomatoes, fresh, diced
2 tbsp chili powder (more or less to taste)
1/2 tsp salt

1. Lightly saute onions and pepper in a non-stick pan over medium heat until slightly soft (3-5 minutes). Add mushrooms and cook 3 minutes more.
2. In a medium stock pot over medium low heat, gently cook diced tomatoes to soften and release their flavor, 15-20 minutes.
3. Brown ground beef, drain from the fat and add beef to the stock pot.
4. Simmer on low heat for about 30 minutes.

Amount Per Serving	
Calories	333.46
Calories From Fat (67%)	223.64

Total Fat 24.24g	
Saturated Fat 9.56g	
Cholesterol 85.05mg	
Sodium 439.88mg	
Potassium 622.71mg	
Total Carbohydrates 6.89g	
Fiber 2.85g	
Sugar 3g	
Protein 21.76g	

67%
7%
26%

KetoHybrid
2014

Broccoli Cheddar Chowder / Cauliflower Chowder

Yield: 4 servings
Serving Size: 1/4 recipe (approximately 9 ounces)
Net Carbs per Serving: 4.7 g
Prep Time: 10 minutes
Cook Time: 15 minutes

1 tbsp onion, minced
1 tbsp butter
1/2 tsp garlic, minced
2 cups fresh broccoli, chopped
3 cups chicken broth
1/2 tsp salt
1/4 tsp black pepper
1/2 cup heavy cream
6 ounces cheddar cheese, grated

Amount Per Serving	
Calories	339.43
Calories From Fat (79%)	267.98

Total Fat 30.36g	
Saturated Fat 18.42g	
Cholesterol 98.29mg	
Sodium 683.46mg	
Potassium 196.58mg	
Total Carbohydrates 4.71g	
Fiber 0.05g	
Sugar 1.12g	
Protein 13.09g	

79%
5%
16%

KetoHybrid
2014

1. In a large stock pot over medium-high heat, heat butter and saute onion, garlic and broccoli until slightly tender (5-7 minutes).
2. Add broth and spices, turn off heat and allow to rest for 5 minutes.
3. Carefully ladle soup to food processor or blender and coarsely blend (not quite a puree).
4. Return soup to the stock pot over low heat and stir in cream.
5. Add cheese and stir until melted.
6. Serve immediately.

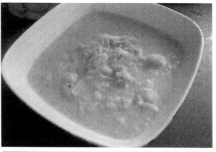

Equally delicious when made with cauliflower (shown at right):

Yield: 4 servings
Serving Size: 1/4 recipe
(approximately 10 ounces)
Net Carbs per Serving: 4.3 g

Amount Per Serving	
Calories	341.99
Calories From Fat (78%)	268.16

Total Fat 30.37g	
Saturated Fat 18.43g	
Cholesterol 98.29mg	
Sodium 688.87mg	
Potassium 230.7mg	
Total Carbohydrates 5.34g	
Fiber 1.05g	
Sugar 2.07g	
Protein 12.99g	

78%
6%
16%

KetoHybrid
2014

CHAPTER 18

Breads & Baked Goods

Breads and baked goods are a large part of the North American diet. Unfortunately they consist primarily of grains (carbohydrates).

It is impossible to perfectly recreate the baked goods you are used to with non-wheat flours. To ensure you don't feel any lack in your diet though we can still make a variety of breads by mixing whole and nutritious foods (seeds, nuts, eggs, etc.).

If you live in the USA you have access to low-carb flours that other countries do not. These products are made with heavily processed and modified ingredients. Many companies selling low-carb products have been caught lying on food labels by the FDA of late[14]. LEARN MORE. (Visit the link or at the very least, perform your own due diligence before buying any pre-made low carb product.)

Your palate will have a lot to do with whether you love the recipes here or not. Each one is a little different in flavor and texture so please try them all before choosing a favorite.

We will be baking with some ingredients that may be unfamiliar to you. They are all available at a large grocery, bulk food, health food store, or online. In comparison to cheap flour, these products will be expensive. Bite for bite though you'll easily be getting ten times the nutrition.

If you already prefer a whole grain bread you'll enjoy these new flavors and textures. Use these recipes as a base for your own creation – suited perfectly to your taste. Add a tablespoon more coconut flour for a finer

---

14 "Low Carb Liars", www.KetoHybrid.com/low-carb-liars

texture. If a recipe turns out too dry for your liking, replace some coconut flour with almond flour. When a recipe doesn't hold together well, add an extra egg (or egg white), some soaked chia seeds, or psyllium. For more texture, add a little extra ground flax seed.

The difference between product brands can vary in texture (grind), fat and moisture content.

One of the most common problems in texture is the mix-up between psyllium husks and psyllium husk powder. I only bake with husks (very inexpensive and beneficial for adding both volume and bind between other ingredients). If you need help with a recipe, let us know.

Finally, if you try a recipe that doesn't turn out to your liking, you don't have to bin it. Cut the bread into cubes and make garlicky croutons, freeze them for a future turkey stuffing, slice and toast the bread for a guilt-free onion soup, or grind the cubes for use as breading.

Croutons & Breadcrumbs

One cup of commercial seasoned bread crumbs contains 82 grams of carbohydrates. One cup of commercial seasoned croutons contains 25 grams of carbohydrates. A cup of bread crumbs or croutons made from these recipes have less than 11 grams of carbohydrates.

To make croutons: Fast fry cubes of bread in coconut oil or butter mixed with your favorite spices. Traditionally this is a light sprinkling of garlic powder and parsley, oregano, or basil.

To make breadcrumbs: Cut or crumble the bread into small pieces and bake on a cookie sheet at 200°F until slightly toasted or dry. Grind in a food processor and store in the freezer until you need them.

Big Chia Dippers

Dippers and crackers can be a challenge on a low carb, high fat diet! We need something for all those yummy cheeses, tzatziki and guacamole, don't we? This cracker is hearty enough for the heaviest dip, low in carbs, and absolutely packed with nutrition! Versatile enough to flavor with your best spices and herbs – complimenting your favorite dip – easily.

Yield: 24 large crackers 2" x 2"
Servings: 6 servings (4 Big Dippers each)
Net Carbs per Serving: 6 grams (1.5 per cracker)
Prep Time: 5 minutes
Bake Time: 1 hour

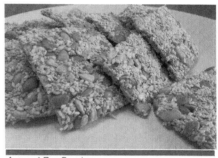

1/2 cup chia seeds
1/2 cup pepitas (pumpkin seeds)
1/2 cup sunflower seeds
1/2 cup sesame seeds, raw
1 cup water
1/2 tsp garlic, freshly minced
1/4 tsp sea salt

Amount Per Serving	
Calories	62.09
Calories From Fat (61%)	37.94

Total Fat 4.53g	
Saturated Fat 0.55g	
Cholesterol 0mg	
Sodium 59.47mg	
Potassium 58.06mg	
Total Carbohydrates 4.19g	
Fiber 2.69g	
Sugar 0.08g	
Protein 2.05g	

61%

11% 27%

KetoHybrid
2014

1. Preheat oven to 325°F. Lightly oil a baking sheet.
2. Mix seeds and garlic together in a medium bowl.
3. Add water and stir until well combined.
4. Spread dipper dough onto baking sheet, evenly pressing it out until approximately 1/4" thick. Reshape edges as necessary.
5. Bake at 325°F for 30 minutes, remove, slice and flip to continue cooking both sides.
6. Return to the oven for another 25-30 minutes or until done.
7. Remove to a wire rack to cool.
8. Store, up to 5 days, in an airy container.

Two, Two Minute English Muffins

Be sure to note the differences in calories and macros between these two. Both are delicious, quick to make, highly functional, and low in carbs but you might prefer one over the other based on your need for dietary fat on any given day.

English Muffin Replacement #1

Yield: 1 muffin to be sliced in half
Serving Size: 1
Net Carbs per Serving: 2 g
Prep Time: 1 minute
Bake Time: 3 minutes including toasting

1 egg
1tsp olive or coconut oil
1 tbsp water
1 tbsp coconut flour
1 tbsp psyllium husks
1 pinch sea salt
1 pinch baking powder

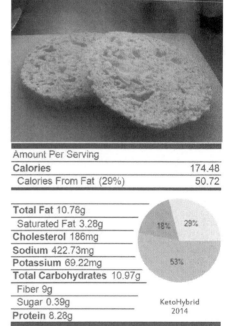

Amount Per Serving	
Calories	174.48
Calories From Fat (29%)	50.72

Total Fat 10.76g	
Saturated Fat 3.28g	
Cholesterol 186mg	
Sodium 422.73mg	
Potassium 69.22mg	
Total Carbohydrates 10.97g	
Fiber 9g	
Sugar 0.39g	
Protein 8.28g	

KetoHybrid
2014

1. In a small glass dish or ramekin, whisk egg with olive oil and water.
2. Whisk in remaining ingredients.
3. Microwave on high for 60-90 seconds.
4. Slice lengthwise, toast, and top with your favorite ingredients.

Large English Muffin #2

Yield: 1 muffin to be sliced in half
Serving Size: 1 muffin
Net Carbs per Serving: 1.7 g
Prep Time: 1 minute
Bake Time: 3 minutes including toasting

1 egg
1 tbsp water
1 tbsp olive or coconut oil
1/3 cup almond flour
2 tbsp golden flax, ground
3/4 tsp baking powder
1 pinch sea salt

1. In a small glass dish or ramekin, whisk egg with olive oil and water.
2. Whisk in remaining ingredients.
3. Microwave on high for two minutes or until the muffin feels firm to the touch.
4. Slice horizontally, toast, and top with your favorite ingredients.

Amount Per Serving	
Calories	368.78
Calories From Fat (77%)	283.87

Total Fat 32.37g	
Saturated Fat 4.31g	77%
Cholesterol 186mg	
Sodium 734.86mg	9%
Potassium 265.01mg	14%
Total Carbohydrates 8.91g	
Fiber 7.22g	
Sugar 0.56g	KetoHybrid
Protein 12.67g	2014

Low Carb Bagels or Bread Loaf

A bagel (or 2 slices from the loaf) measure in at just 5.6 net carbs. Compare that to an average grocery store bagel; 55 carbs, 8 g fiber, 47 net carbs (yes forty-seven).

Yield: 10 bagels or 1 loaf (cut into 20 slices)
Serving Size: 1 bagel or two slices of bread
Net Carbs per Serving: 2.8 grams
Prep Time: 10 minutes
Bake Time: 30 minutes

1 1/2 cups almond flour
1/4 cup flax seed, ground
2 tbsp chickpea flour (basan)
1 tsp baking soda
1/4 tsp sea salt
5 eggs
2 tbsp apple cider vinegar

Topping variations: 1 tbsp sesame seeds, poppy seeds, garlic powder, finely diced onion

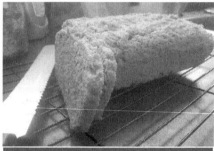

Amount Per Serving	
Calories	128.39
Calories From Fat (64%)	82.71
Total Fat 9.81g	
Saturated Fat 1.01g	
Cholesterol 37.2mg	
Sodium 201.44mg	
Potassium 171.64mg	
Total Carbohydrates 5.93g	
Fiber 3.1g	
Sugar 0.97g	
Protein 5.62g	

64%

19%

16%

KetoHybrid
2014

1. Preheat oven to 350°F. Lightly oil a non-stick pan with coconut oil. Bagels are made in an oiled, non-stick donut pan.
2. In a large bowl or food processor, mix dry ingredients.
3. Add whole eggs and apple cider vinegar and continue mixing for 3-4 minutes.
4. The dough will be thinner than a standard bread dough but not as thin as a cake batter. This dough will double in size during baking.
5. Bake for 17-20 minutes (bagels), 30 minutes (loaf).
6. Bagels and bread freeze well – slice before freezing for ease of use. Defrost at room temperature.

No Corn Cornbread

Moist, filling, and KetoHybrid approved! You can cook this in the oven, on the grill, and even in a microwave if you're short on time. Goes beautifully with our Pulled Pork Recipe or Bean-Free Chili.

If you like your cornbread with something a little extra – garlic powder, chopped chili, or cheddar cheese – feel free to add to this recipe. I've been known to leave out the onions and add homemade chunky applesauce for a sweet treat. Anything goes as long as it isn't corn! (Adjust nutrition for your additions.)

Yield: Eight 1″ squares
Serving Size: One 1″ square
Net Carbs per Serving: 0.6 grams
Prep Time: 5 minutes
Bake Time: 20 minutes (oven), 15 minutes (grill), 6 minutes (microwave)

2 eggs, lightly beaten
2 tbsp butter, melted but not hot
1/4 cup sour cream
1 cup almond flour
1/4 cup green onions, diced (both white and green sections, approximately 2 onions)
3/4 tsp baking powder
1/4 tsp sea salt

1. Preheat oven to 350°F. Lightly oil a square baking dish if cooking in the oven; a 12" cast iron pan if grilling, or a 10" glass pie plate if cooking in the microwave. We own a low-powered microwave and needed to cook this in two equal batches for even heat distribution.
2. In a medium bowl, combine beaten eggs, butter and sour cream until combined. Add remaining ingredients.
3. Pour batter into pan and bake for 20 minutes or until top is golden brown.
4. Serve immediately or store in refrigerator up to one week.

Amount Per Serving	
Calories	76.41
Calories From Fat (82%)	62.38

Total Fat 6.99g	
Saturated Fat 3.04g	
Cholesterol 57.87mg	
Sodium 142.77mg	
Potassium 36.96mg	
Total Carbohydrates 0.9g	
Fiber 0.33g	
Sugar 0.37g	
Protein 2.56g	

82%
4%
14%

KetoHybrid
2014

Golden Flax Wraps

This recipe was a lifesaver when we first started our KetoHybrid diet! We barely noticed that we weren't getting all our carbs as these wraps are similar in taste to whole wheat flax wraps.

These are twice as filling as a grocery store wrap and are perfect for burritos, quesadillas (two wraps held together by a thick cheddar cheese filling, then warmed in a hot skillet) and breakfast wraps.

If you use a standard ground flax seed – instead of golden – the resulting wrap is tough and less pliable.

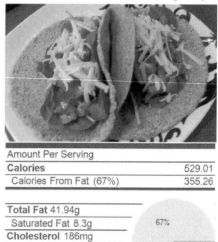

Yield: Five 7" wraps

Serving Size: 1 wrap

Net Carbs per Serving: 2.5 net carbs

Prep Time: 2 minutes

Bake Time: 10 minutes (oven); or 3-4 minutes (microwave)

2 cups golden flax seeds, ground

4 eggs

4 tsp coconut oil, warmed to liquid state

4 tbsp water

1 tsp baking soda

1 1/2 tsp onion powder

1 1/2 tsp garlic powder

1/2 tsp sea salt

Amount Per Serving	
Calories	529.01
Calories From Fat (67%)	355.26

Total Fat 41.94g		
Saturated Fat 8.3g		67%
Cholesterol 186mg		
Sodium 700.94mg		18%
Potassium 716.11mg		15%
Total Carbohydrates 23.82g		
Fiber 21.31g		
Sugar 1.43g		KetoHybrid
Protein 20.68g		2014

1. Mix dry ingredients in a medium bowl.
2. Mix eggs, oil, water in a small bowl.
3. Stir egg mixture into the dry mix until a consistent texture is achieved. The mixture will be thick, but not dry. If it doesn't appear to be spreadable, mix in another tablespoon of water.
4. Lightly oil a glass pie plate with olive or coconut oil.
5. Add 1/2 cup of mixture to the pie plate. Gently spread it with the back of a spoon or spatula to fill the bottom of the plate.
6. Cook until the center has cooked through – on high in microwave for 2 1/2 - 3 1/2 minutes each, or in a preheated 350°F oven for 10 minutes.
7. Remove from the pan and serve.

Eat A Muffin Top, Lose The Muffin Top

Got a hankering for banana bread? These muffin tops will quiet those beastly cravings. We decreased net carbs to just 6 grams, a great feat when compared to a slice from a traditional loaf of banana bread (32 net carbs).

There are multiple ways to make a banana muffin with fewer carbs, but they omit the actual banana by using a flavored protein powder or a flavor extracts. Most protein powders and flavor extracts contain questionable ingredients. On the other hand, real bananas offer many nutrients that may be missing in your diet so indulge; each muffin contains 1/3 of a real banana.

Yield: 12 muffin tops
Serving Size: 1 muffin top
Net Carbs per Serving: 6 grams
Prep Time: 5-10 minutes
Bake Time: 20 minutes

1 1/2 cup almond flour
1 tsp baking soda
1 1/4 cup mashed bananas (about 4 medium bananas)
1 egg, beaten
1/4 cup butter, melted
1 tbsp sugar substitute (easily omitted)

Crumble Top:
2 tbsp almond flour
1/4 tsp ground cinnamon
1 tbsp butter

Amount Per Serving	
Calories	143.32
Calories From Fat (69%)	99.56
Total Fat 11.63g	
Saturated Fat 3.67g	
Cholesterol 28.21mg	
Sodium 160.26mg	
Potassium 182.01mg	
Total Carbohydrates 8.22g	
Fiber 2.21g	
Sugar 3.39g	
Protein 3.56g	

69%
22%
9%

KetoHybrid
2014

1. Preheat oven to 350°F.
2. Liberally oil a non-stick muffin top baking pan.
3. In a medium sized bowl, mix almond flour and baking soda.
4. In a separate bowl: first mash bananas, then add egg and melted butter.
5. Add wet mixture to dry. Stir until just combined.
6. Measure 1/4 cup batter into each muffin top slot.
7. Mix crumble ingredients together and distribute evenly across the tops of muffins.
8. Bake for 15-18 minutes or until tops are golden brown.

Blueberry Muffins

Yield: 10 muffins

Serving Size: 1 muffin

Net Carbs per Serving: 3.7 grams

Prep Time: 10 minutes

Bake Time: 20 minutes

2 cups almond flour

1/2 tsp baking soda

1/2 tsp baking powder

1/8 tsp salt

1 cup blueberries

3 eggs, beaten

1/4 cup coconut oil, melted

1 tbsp sugar substitute (easily omitted)

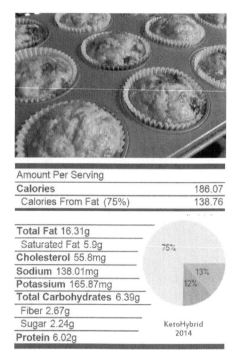

Amount Per Serving	
Calories	186.07
Calories From Fat (75%)	138.76

Total Fat 16.31g	
Saturated Fat 5.9g	
Cholesterol 55.8mg	
Sodium 138.01mg	
Potassium 165.87mg	
Total Carbohydrates 6.39g	
Fiber 2.67g	
Sugar 2.24g	
Protein 6.02g	

KetoHybrid
2014

1. Preheat oven to 325°F. Lightly oil a non-stick muffin pan.
2. In a medium sized bowl, mix almond flour, baking soda, baking powder, salt and sugar substitute (if using).
3. In a separate bowl: beat eggs and continue to whisk while slowly drizzling in the warmed coconut oil. The coconut oil may solidify into small clumps while whisking due to the coldness of the eggs. Any small clumps will disperse during baking.
4. Add wet mixture to dry and stir until just combined. Fold in blueberries.
5. Measure an approximate 1/3 cup batter for each muffin.
6. Bake for 18-20 minutes or until tops are golden brown.
7. Individually wrapped, these freeze well up to 2 weeks.

Lemon Poppy Seed Muffins

A subtle lemon poppy seed muffin that, when baked with honey, are still relatively low in calories and net carbs. Substitute honey with an artificial sweetener if you like and you'll have a zesty morning muffin just over 1 gram of net carbs.

Compare the KetoHybrid Lemon Poppy Seed Muffins!
Donut Shop Muffin (15% larger in volume): 510 calories and 79 g net carbs.
KetoHybrid Muffin, honey: 130 calories and 4.8 g net carbs.
KetoHybrid Muffin, artificial sweetener: 117 calories and 1.1 g net carbs.

Yield: 10 muffins
Serving Size: 1 muffin
Net Carbs per Serving: 4.8 grams (honey); 1.1 grams (sugar substitute)
Prep Time: 10 minutes
Bake Time: 20 minutes

1/2 cup of coconut flour
1/2 tsp of sea salt
1/4 tsp of baking soda
4 eggs
1/3 cup coconut oil
2 tbsp honey
1 tsp vanilla
1 tbsp poppy seeds
1 tbsp lemon zest

Amount Per Serving	
Calories	129.81
Calories From Fat (69%)	89.02
Total Fat 10.23g	
Saturated Fat 7.65g	69%
Cholesterol 74.4mg	
Sodium 186.31mg	
Potassium 37.72mg	
Total Carbohydrates 7g	
Fiber 2.18g	
Sugar 3.8g	KetoHybrid
Protein 3.13g	2014

1. Preheat oven to 350°F. Lightly oil a non-stick muffin pan.
2. In a medium sized bowl, mix coconut flour, salt, baking soda, poppy seeds, and sugar substitute (if using).
3. In a separate bowl: beat eggs and continue to whisk while slowly drizzling in the warmed coconut oil, vanilla extract, lemon zest and honey (if using).
4. The coconut oil may solidify into small clumps while whisking due to the coldness of the eggs. Those small clumps will disperse during baking.
5. Add wet mixture to dry. Stir until just combined.
6. Measure an approximate 1/3 cup batter for each muffin.
7. Bake for 18-20 minutes or until tops are golden brown.
8. Individually wrapped, these freeze well up to 2 weeks.
   Nutrition shown for version made with honey.

Rosemary and Garlic Artisan Crackers

Great for scooping guacamole! The photo shows the crackers made with regular ground flax seeds. Substitute golden ground flax seeds for a lighter texture and color.

Leftovers can be stored on the counter in a large plastic or glass container for 2-3 days. They've never lasted any longer in our house – just because they're such a popular nibbler.

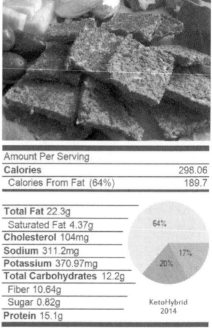

Amount Per Serving	
Calories	298.06
Calories From Fat (64%)	189.7

Yield: About 80 small crackers (1"x1")

Serving Size: 1/4 recipe or 20 crackers

Net Carbs per Serving: 1.6

Prep Time: 15 minutes

Bake Time: 15 minutes

Total Fat 22.3g	
Saturated Fat 4.37g	64%
Cholesterol 104mg	
Sodium 311.2mg	
Potassium 370.97mg	17%
Total Carbohydrates 12.2g	20%
Fiber 10.64g	
Sugar 0.82g	KetoHybrid
Protein 15.1g	2014

1 cup flax seeds, ground

2 eggs

1/2 cup Parmesan cheese, freshly grated

1 tsp dried rosemary, ground

1/2 tsp garlic powder

1/8 tsp sea salt (for tops, optional, included in nutrition data)

1. Preheat oven to 350°F. Lightly oil a large baking sheet or silicone baking mat.
2. Add all ingredients to a medium bowl and stir until combined. Let sit for 5 minutes.
3. This dough needs to be rolled out 1/4 – 1/8" thickness. It will stick to your counter so roll it out between two sheets of parchment paper, wax paper, or some well-oiled saran wrap.
4. Cut rolled dough into a grid of 1"-2" in squares or rectangles. Bake directly on parchment paper or transfer the cut dough individually to a baking sheet or silicone mat. No space is required between the crackers while baking.
5. Salt lightly and place in the oven for 10 minutes. Remove from oven, flip crackers and continue baking for another 3-5 minutes.

Whole Wheat Bread or Rolls

We've only make this recipe once past perfecting it because we've now lost the cravings for yeast-risen breads. You may as well, but if not, this recipe tastes as good as any high-grain, grocery store loaf.

The average slice of a heavy whole grain bread has 20 grams carbs, 17 net carbs and 110 calories. This version has 5.6 grams carb, 3.3 grams net carbs and 84 calories per slice.

Makes 15 dinner rolls, 2 small loaves, or one full size loaf. In the photo you can see that I made 2 small loaves but had to cut them horizontally to have a standard-sized slice. From that batch I ended up with 16 slices total, but one of the top slices went straight to the bread crumbs bag (it was broken and thin).

Yield: 15 rolls or slices of bread (baked in one large or two small loaves)
Serving Size: one slice
Net Carbs per Serving: 3.3 grams
Prep Time: 15-20 minutes
Bake Time: 30-45 minutes

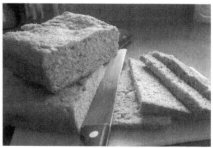

3/4 cup warm water
1 tbsp olive oil
1 1/2 tsp rapid-rise yeast

3/4 cup almond flour
3/4 cup wheat bran, lightly toasted
2/3 cups vital wheat gluten*
1/3 cup whole-wheat flour, stone ground
1/4 tsp sea salt
coconut oil or butter

1. Preheat oven to 150°F and turn off. This will be your rising oven, still warm enough after mixing and shaping your dough.
2. Lightly oil bread pans, muffin tins or a baking sheet with coconut oil or butter.
3. In a large bowl or food processor, gently combine the first three ingredients. Rest for 5 minutes to activate yeast.
4. In a separate bowl, mix remaining dry ingredients.
5. Mix dry ingredients into the wet and knead for 5 minutes. You're looking for perfect dough consistency which can be elusive if measurements are

slightly off. The dough should hold together as a ball – neither runny nor crumbly. Adjust consistency by adding up to a tablespoon of warm water or a tablespoon of whole wheat flour.

6. Shape dough into loaves or buns and lightly oil the tops.
7. Place loaves or buns into the still warm oven, to rise for one hour - 2-3 times in volume.
8. Leaving loaves or buns in the oven, turn the oven to 350°F and bake for 30-40 minutes.
9. Cool on a wire rack before slicing.

*Nutrition Data: I'm not certain that Vital Wheat Gluten macro-nutrients are consistent worldwide. Calculation is based on a weight of 5.5 dry ounces per cup.

Amount Per Serving	
Calories	83.97
Calories From Fat (55%)	45.8
Total Fat 5.36g	
Saturated Fat 1.92g	
Cholesterol 0mg	
Sodium 40.78mg	
Potassium 85.84mg	
Total Carbohydrates 5.6g	
Fiber 2.24g	
Sugar 0.21g	
Protein 5.31g	

55%

23%

KetoHybrid
2014

KetoHybrid Bun

Hearty enough to hold a burger with all your favorite condiments. At their best when lightly toasted.

Follow the recipe for dinner or burger buns, or omit the garlic/onion powder for your nut butter eaters – they're great toasted, then slathered with nut butter.

Yield: 5 hamburger-size buns (shape them into 10 buns for sliders)
Serving Size: 1 hamburger sized bun
Net Carbs per Serving: 2.9 grams
Prep Time: 10 minutes
Bake Time: 45 minutes

3/4 cup almond flour
1/4 cup psyllium husks
1/3 cup coconut flour
1/4 cup ground flax seed (regular or golden)
1 tsp cream of tartar
1/2 tsp baking soda
3 large egg whites
1 large free-range egg
1 tsp garlic powder
1 tsp onion powder
1 cup boiling water
1/3 tsp salt
2 1/2 tbsp sesame seeds

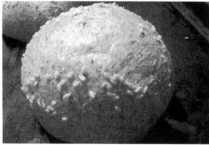

1. Preheat the oven to 350°F.
2. In a large bowl or food processor, mix all dry ingredients except for sesame seeds.
3. Add egg whites and whole egg. Mix well until the dough is thick and well blended.
4. Add boiling water and continue to mix on a dough setting (food processor), or low (hand mixer) for another 2-3 minutes. The dough should start to firm up a little at this time.
5. Split dough into 5 equal portions. With moist hands, shape and smooth each portion and place on a non-stick baking tray. Provide ample space between each bun, they will triple in size.
6. Top each with 10-12 sesame seeds before baking.

7. Bake for at least 40 minutes (45 if you have opened the oven door). Buns will have fully risen after 20 minutes but don't take them out too early or they will fall.

Amount Per Serving	
Calories	146.7
Calories From Fat (33%)	47.99

Total Fat 7.48g	
Saturated Fat 1.75g	
Cholesterol 37.2mg	
Sodium 334.3mg	
Potassium 242.13mg	
Total Carbohydrates 13.36g	
Fiber 10.46g	
Sugar 0.5g	
Protein 6.48g	

33%
18%
49%

KetoHybrid
2014

CHAPTER 19

Eggs & Breakfast Recipes

One of our most eaten breakfast recipes are a low carb high fat breakfast sandwich. Dependent on what's in our cupboard we make one of the (less than 1 net carb) English muffin replacement, fry an egg, warm up a sausage patty and top with cheese. You can eat them on the road when you're rushed or make them ahead of time for a workday lunch.

Be sure to check out other sections of this book for more breakfast ideas:

In Entrees: Scotch Eggs
In Sauces: Hollandaise, Any Berry Syrup, Jam
In Breads: Low Carb Bagel, One Minute Breakfast Sandwich Bun, Muffins
In Desserts: Blueberry Scones, 3 Minute Muffin

KetoHybrid Classic Breakfast Sandwich

The two KetoHybrid sandwiches below contain the same 'stack' but use different buns – both recipes are in the breads chapter. Note that net carbs per sandwich are the same, their macros are quite different. Choose based on your expected meals for the day.

Variation #1

Yield: 1 sandwich

Serves: 1

Net Carbs per serving: 3.7 g

Prep Time: 5 minutes

Cook Time: 5 minutes

1 sausage patty (1 ounce)

1 egg

2 oz cheddar cheese

1 English Muffin Replacement #1 (coconut flour version)

1. Fry or poach one egg, ensuring that the yolk is fully cooked.
2. Make English muffin Replacement #1, halve horizontally and toast.
3. Warm one pre-cooked, homemade sausage patty (recipe on next page).
4. Assemble sandwich.

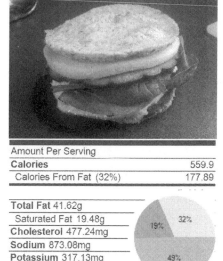

Amount Per Serving	
Calories	559.9
Calories From Fat (32%)	177.89

Total Fat 41.62g	
Saturated Fat 19.48g	
Cholesterol 477.24mg	
Sodium 873.08mg	
Potassium 317.13mg	
Total Carbohydrates 10.68g	
Fiber 7.03g	
Sugar 0.93g	
Protein 34.97g	

KetoHybrid 2014

Variation #2

Yield: 1 sandwich

Serves: 1

Net Carbs per serving: 3.7 g

Prep Time: 5 minutes

Cook Time: 5 minutes

Same as above but using English Muffin Replacement #2 (almond flour version)

Amount Per Serving	
Calories	765.54
Calories From Fat (73%)	557.95

Total Fat 63.24g	
Saturated Fat 20.5g	
Cholesterol 477.24mg	
Sodium 1185.21mg	
Potassium 512.91mg	
Total Carbohydrates 11.3g	
Fiber 7.59g	
Sugar 1.1g	
Protein 39.36g	

KetoHybrid 2014

Sausage Patties

Yield: 8 one-ounce patties
Serving Size: 1 patty
Net Carbs per serving: 0.6 g
Prep Time: 5 minutes
Cook Time: 5 minutes

1 pound ground pork
1 tbsp garlic, minced
1 egg
1 tsp cumin
1 tsp oregano
1/4 tsp cayenne
1/4 tsp black pepper
1/4 tsp salt

1. Mix all ingredients together, divide and shape into 8 thin patties, approximately 4" in diameter.
2. Fry over medium-high heat, 3-4 minutes per side, or until cooked through.
3. Serve immediately or cool on a wire rack before storage.
4. Store in the refrigerator up to one week, or freezer up to 2 months. Freeze stacks of patties with a small piece of wax paper between each for easy access.

Amount Per Serving	
Calories	161.84
Calories From Fat (71%)	114.35
Total Fat 12.69g	
Saturated Fat 4.67g	71%
Cholesterol 64.07mg	
Sodium 41.37mg	2%
Potassium 185.68mg	28%
Total Carbohydrates 0.8g	
Fiber 0.17g	
Sugar 0.06g	KetoHybrid
Protein 10.52g	2014

Florentine Baked Eggs

This fast and delicious egg dish is easily scaled up or down, looks fancier than 'yet another omelet' and suits any meal. These were made in heart shaped ramekins.

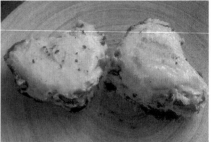

Yield: 2 ramekins
Serving Size: Full Recipe
Net Carbs per Serving: 3.6 grams
Prep Time: 10 minutes
Cook Time: 10-12 minutes

1 tbsp butter
1 cup fresh spinach leaves, coarsely chopped
1/4 cup ricotta cheese (full fat version)
2 tbsp Parmesan cheese, grated and divided
2 large eggs
1/2 tsp salt
1/8 tsp white pepper

1. Preheat oven to 350°F. Lightly oil two ovenproof ramekins.
2. Add butter and spinach to a small frying pan and lightly saute over medium-high heat until spinach slightly wilts. Turn off the heat, mix in ricotta, half the Parmesan, salt and pepper.
3. Divide spinach and cheese mixture between the two ramekins – shaping part of the mixture up sides of ramekins.
4. Crack one whole egg onto each spinach 'nest'. Top with final tablespoon Parmesan.
5. Bake until set – 10 minutes for a slightly soft egg, 12 for a firmer egg.
6. Serve directly in ramekins or invert onto a plate.

Amount Per Serving	
Calories	402.71
Calories From Fat (70%)	283.27

Total Fat 31.99g	
Saturated Fat 17.27g	70%
Cholesterol 442.7mg	
Sodium 1534.58mg	4%
Potassium 386.34mg	26%
Total Carbohydrates 4.3g	
Fiber 0.74g	
Sugar 0.76g	KetoHybrid
Protein 24.34g	2014

Speedy Savory Muffins

The easiest, low carb breakfast known to mom. Once a week we make 6-12 of these and leave them in the refrigerator for rushed or lazy mornings. Heat one up – breakfast is served and they travel well for work lunches too!

The most basic version of this recipe follows. Add in your favorite vegetables, swap out meats and cheese, anything goes as long as you adjust your carb counts and are aware of your macros throughout the day. Leftover cauliflower, broccoli, mushrooms, spinach and small amounts of red pepper work well when beaten into the egg.

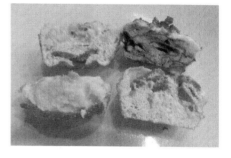

Yield: 6 muffins
Serving Size: 1 of 6 muffins
Net Carbs per serving: 1.3 grams
Prep Time: 10 minutes
Cook Time: 15 minutes

6 slices bacon*, cooked
6 eggs
1 tbsp butter
3 ounces Swiss cheese, cut into six equal portions
1 pinch onion powder

1. Preheat oven to 375°F. Lightly oil a non-stick muffin pan.
2. Place one slice of meat in the bottom of each muffin cup.
3. Gently beat eggs with onion powder (plus any extra vegetables or spices).
4. Pour egg mixture over meat, evenly between the six muffin cups.
5. Bake for 10-12 minutes or until the egg has set.
6. Top each muffin with a half slice of cheese. Return to the oven to soften the cheese (1-2 minutes).
7. Serve immediately or allow to cool before storage.

Nutrition calculated for 1/3 pound bacon. Bacon thickness varies by brand and butcher. An average 1/3 pound of bacon is roughly equivalent to 6 slices, medium thick.

Amount Per Serving	
Calories	180.63
Calories From Fat (67%)	120.92
Total Fat 13.56g	
Saturated Fat 6.27g	67%
Cholesterol 211.88mg	
Sodium 358.23mg	3%
Potassium 120.8mg	30%
Total Carbohydrates 1.26g	
Fiber 0.01g	
Sugar 0.38g	KetoHybrid
Protein 12.73g	2014

Low Carb High Fat Eggs Benedict

Little else fits with a lazy Sunday morning than a plate of Eggs Benedict made with fresh, free range eggs purchased the day before at the Farmer's Market. They look impressive, taste divine, and increase your fat intake!

For the cook they are a masterpiece of timing unless the prep work was performed a day before. Get out of the kitchen quicker with cooked bacon and Hollandaise sauce on hand. Thin-sliced, low carb buns replace traditional English Muffins – all you need to do is lightly toast them and get stacking!

Yield: 4 servings

Serving Size: 2 eggs per person

Net Carbs per Serving: 5.7 g per serving

Prep Time: 20 minutes

Cook Time: 15 minutes

8 slices of peameal bacon, cooked (1 ounce per slice)

8 eggs

1 cup Blender Hollandaise (recipe in sauces)

1 avocado, sliced*

4-6 leaves Boston or Bib lettuce, or baby spinach

4 low carb English Muffin Replacement #1, split and toasted (recipe in breads)

Amount Per Serving	
Calories	613.83
Calories From Fat (74%)	451.9

Total Fat 51.49g		
Saturated Fat 21.58g	74%	
Cholesterol 596.59mg		
Sodium 1103.33mg	6%	
Potassium 590.16mg	21%	
Total Carbohydrates 9.27g		
Fiber 4.62g		
Sugar 0.73g	KetoHybrid	
Protein 30.27g	2014	

1. Gently crack 8 eggs into a poaching pan and cook until the yolk has firmed but is still slightly soft.
2. While eggs are cooking, warm Hollandaise and bacon, lightly toast buns, and slice avocado.
3. Make your Benedict stacks, two per plate: half bun, small lettuce leaf, peameal slice, avocado slice, one egg, 1/4 cup of Hollandaise sauce.
4. Garnish with a sprinkling of parsley, some freshly ground black pepper and serve.

- Omit avocado to decrease 71 calories and 1.4 net carbs per serving.

Fast Fast Frittata

A perfectly fast and delicious meal that uses up any cooked vegetable in your fridge. We almost always have cooked cauliflower and fresh spinach in the fridge but fritattas taste great with every vegetable.

Yield: 10" frittata

Serving Size: 1/2 recipe

Net Carbs per serving: 2.2 g

Prep Time: 10 minutes

Cook Time: 15 minutes

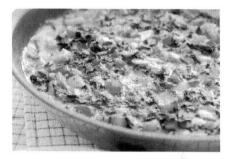

4 eggs

2 tbsp coconut oil (or butter)

1/4 cup cream, half & half

1/3 cup fresh spinach, coarsely chopped

1/3 cup cauliflower, cooked and coarsely chopped

1/4 cup sweet red pepper, diced

1/8 tsp onion powder

1/8 tsp salt

1/8 tsp black pepper, freshly ground

1. Melt butter or coconut oil in an oven-safe skillet over medium heat. Add all vegetables and lightly saute until warmed through.
2. Whisk 4 eggs with the cream in a medium bowl and add to the frying pan. Turn heat to medium-low.
3. When the eggs have set on the sides and bottom, split the frittata in two and flip each side directly in the pan, or place the pan under your oven's broiler for 3-4 minutes.
4. Serve with a tablespoon of sugar free, home made salsa, if desired (adjust carbs).

Amount Per Serving	
Calories	309.27
Calories From Fat (76%)	234.3

Total Fat 26.7g	
Saturated Fat 17.07g	
Cholesterol 383.19mg	
Sodium 309.28mg	
Potassium 282.5mg	
Total Carbohydrates 3.93g	
Fiber 0.74g	
Sugar 1.25g	
Protein 14.06g	

76%

5%

19%

KetoHybrid
2014

No Oats Oatmeal

This breakfast bowl is quick and basic. You're invited to add variety to the pot once it gets cooking. My Scottish heritage makes me want chopped nuts, fruits, and whole seeds in oatmeal. This is still satisfying even without added fruit. Use spices to add even more variety, such as nutmeg, cloves or cardamom. Top with a little cream, almond milk or coconut milk if that's how you prefer regular oatmeal.

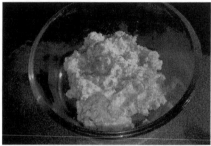

Yields: 3/4 - 1 cup

Serves: 1

Net Carbs per serving: 2.8 g

Prep Time: 0 minutes

Cook Time: 5 minutes

2 eggs

1/3 cup cream (works just as well with almond or coconut milk)

1 tbsp coconut flour

1 tbsp butter

1/2 tsp cinnamon

1/8 tsp vanilla extract

1. In a small saucepan over medium heat, beat eggs and cream. Whisk in remaining ingredients and keep whisking until the mixture reaches the consistency of coarse cooked oatmeal.
2. Add butter to the saucepan and continue to gently stir and cook the "no oats oatmeal" for another minute.
3. Serve as is, with a few tablespoons of cream (adjust nutrition using the counts provided in this book), or with a sprinkling of sugar substitute.

Amount Per Serving	
Calories	199.17
Calories From Fat (31%)	62.01

Total Fat 15.91g	
Saturated Fat 8.65g	
Cholesterol 216.17mg	
Sodium 138.3mg	
Potassium 126.29mg	
Total Carbohydrates 5.65g	
Fiber 2.9g	
Sugar 0.4g	
Protein 8.56g	

31%

18%

0%

51%

KetoHybrid
2014

CHAPTER 20

Entrees & Dinner Ideas

Dinners, in my opinion, are the easiest dietary change to make. I'm going to assume that you already have a large repetoire of dinner favorites. If so, you should carry on making those dishes with the omission of starchy accompaniments.

If your menu looks like ours once did – meat, starch, vegetable – you'll need some ideas on replacing pasta, rice and potatoes. Don't worry, we've got you covered!

Noodle Alternatives

For dishes that traditionally require pasta noodles, substitute with zucchini noodles for a nutritious and low carb alternative. If your sauce is flavorful and you haven't over-cooked the zucchini, you'll fall in love with this simple easy swap. In the beginning of my low-carb journey I would peel, then julienne, then salt and drain (to remove extra moisture), and finally cook, the zucchini. I have tried fast fry, roasting, dehydration, and cooking in the microwave for this noodle alternative. While I'm not a fan of microwave ovens, I won't lie to you; 2-3 minutes on high provides the best results.

Finally, it won't be long before you're frustrated by the time it takes to cut thin strips of zucchini by hand – no matter how good it tastes – especially if you are cooking meals for more than one person. For less than $20 you can

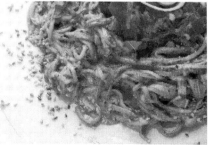

purchase a small tool that quickly and easily turns zucchini into long, consistently sized, noodles. I bought mine at the Farmer's Market but they are available online[15], for less money. The dish below was made with the thick side of my spiralizer, olive oil, chopped tomatoes, fresh basil and a few sesame seeds.

There are other noodle options – spaghetti squash and hiratimi (find the proper name) noodles for instance – but not everyone has a palate that appreciates those two items.

In my opinion, the flavor and texture of Spaghetti squash overpowers most dishes and doesn't fool anyone. The shiratki noodles are expensive and often very salty. Try each of them once, just so you know what you're not missing.

Rice Alternative

There really is only one acceptable substitute – riced cauliflower. One cup of cooked rice = carbs. One cup of cooked cauliflower = carbs.

I rice my cauliflower in a food processor – both florets and the stalk. This takes 2 minutes of preparation time, then 5-7 minutes to cook (microwave).

You can make any of your favorite rice dishes using cauliflower as long as you're not adding carb-laden beans or sweet sauces to the dish.

Ground Beef – So Much More Than A Burger

Any cut of grass fed beef is expensive, so if your budget is tight buy ground beef and experiment with the many ways of serving it. If you have a good source for organically grown turkey, chicken, or pork, and would rather use those in your recipes, by all means do so.

Here are rough estimates of each, per pound, cooked:

- 80% lean ground beef – 805 calories, 52 grams fat, 80 grams protein
- ground chicken – 284 calories, 17 grams fat, 35 grams protein
- ground turkey – 348 calories, 20 grams fat, 41 grams protein

---

15 www.KetoHybrid.com/spiralizer

- ground pork – 445 calories, 32 grams fat, 39 grams protein

Our family of four purchases between 6-9 pounds per week from the local butcher. I immediately set to work making meatballs of various sizes, then cook them all at once, freezing what I won't be using in the next few days' meals. Meatballs go in soups, make great mid-day snacks, can be layered with zucchini and cheese like a lasagna, or served as is.

During the summer months we are naturally drawn to spending more time by the barbeque; enjoying our burgers. Again, we buy our week's needs, make up a batch of burgers and freeze them.

If you've ever been in a gathering of low carb dieters you'd think that a hamburger was as dull as dust. Even low carb high fat dieters have been known to whine, "If I have to eat one more hamburger slathered in mayonnaise, I'll scream!"

Burgers never get boring – as long as you have a few extra ingredients and a little imagination you can eat hamburgers every night for a month and not get bored. Here are some ideas to get you started:

1. Mix in some pesto for a slightly nutty Mediterranean flavor.
2. Make it Greek! Mix feta cheese and chopped black olives into your ground beef and serve with KetoHybrid's Tzatziki Sauce.
3. Deep South burgers have grated gruyere cheese, grainy Dijon mustard and chopped pecans mixed in. Top that with mayo and you'll never say a burger is boring again.
4. Make a "meatza burger" by topping a cooked hamburger with a 1/2 teaspoon of pizza sauce, 2 ounces of mozzarella and a few slices of pepperoni.
5. Place it under the broiler for a few minutes until the cheese bubbles and browns slightly.
6. Simply Blue, is a burger that merely has an ounce of blue cheese melting on top. So easy, and so delicious; even if you don't like blue cheese.
7. Stuffed burgers – your favorite toppings, hidden inside. Form the patty around some cooked bacon and cheddar cheese, or mushrooms and swiss, or whatever else you can dream up.
8. The Klondike – we used to serve these at a restaurant I worked at 30 years ago. A hamburger patty topped with cooked peameal

bacon (also known as Canadian Bacon) and a few ounces of Hollandaise sauce.

Make Ahead Meatballs

With the right spices and in various sizes meatballs are also made more interesting. One of our favorite (and quickest) dinners is a homemade bone broth soup with leftover vegetables and pre-cooked mini meatballs. With soup stock and mini meatballs waiting in the freezer, dinner is ready in less than twenty minutes. (Before serving add a small handful of fresh spinach and 1/2 teaspoon of freshly grated Parmesan cheese per bowl.)

Extra large meatballs are fun as well. Try wrapping 2-3 ounces of ground beef (between a golf ball and tennis ball in size) around a 1/2" cube of cheese. Best eaten on the day you cook them as some cheese always manages to escape onto the baking sheet.

One pound of of ground beef will make approximately 16 average (1" inch diameter) meatballs. A basic recipe follows but please experiment with your favorite herbs, spices, and saucy toppings. As always, remember to adjust the nutrition counts to reflect your changes.

Cold Beef Dinner Salad

Put that extra steak you barbequed last night in this delicious entree salad for two! It provides great nutrition and is substantial enough to please even the hungriest and hard working.

Yield: 2 entree salads
Serving Size: 3 cups salad that includes 4 ounces of beef
Net Carbs per Serving: 5.7 grams
Prep Time: 20 minutes

4 cups tender lettuce leaves
8 ounces cold sirloin steak, sliced thin (or deli sliced roast beef with no additives)
1/4 cup sweet red bell pepper, cut into thin strips
1/4 cup red onion, sliced thin
1/2 cup parsley, chopped
1/2 cup mushrooms, raw, sliced thin

Salad Dressing:
1/4 cup olive oil
1/8 cup white vinegar
1 tbsp mayonnaise (preferably KetoHybrid Mayo)
1/4 tsp garlic, fresh, minced
1/2 tsp black pepper
1/2 tsp salt

1. In a small bowl, mix dressing ingredients together.
2. Arrange remaining ingredients on two large dinner plates.
3. Top with salad dressing and enjoy!

Amount Per Serving	
Calories	503.97
Calories From Fat (70%)	352.02
Total Fat 39.65g	
Saturated Fat 7.73g	70%
Cholesterol 82.91mg	
Sodium 712.62mg	
Potassium 757.58mg	
Total Carbohydrates 8.68g	
Fiber 2.98g	
Sugar 1.85g	KetoHybrid
Protein 29.23g	2014

Ground Beef Meatballs

Yield: 4 Servings
Serving size: Four 1" meatballs
Net Carbs per Serving: 0.4 g
Prep Time: 5 minutes
Cook Time: 20 minutes

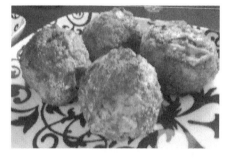

1 lb ground beef, regular
1 egg
1 tsp oregano
1 tsp parsley flakes
1/2 tsp salt
1/2 tsp garlic powder
1/2 tsp thyme

1. Preheat oven to 400°F.
2. In a medium bowl, mix together all ingredients.
3. Form 16 1" balls and place on baking sheet.
4. Bake for approximately 20 minutes.
5. Serve immediately, refrigerate leftovers, or freeze up to one month.

Amount Per Serving	
Calories	320.12
Calories From Fat (71%)	227.87

Total Fat 24.66g	
Saturated Fat 9.83g	71%
Cholesterol 131.55mg	
Sodium 387.28mg	
Potassium 325.81mg	28%
Total Carbohydrates 0.76g	
Fiber 0.27g	
Sugar 0.08g	KetoHybrid
Protein 21.75g	2014

KetoHybrid Shepherd's Pie

A simple and hearty meal made healthier by the omission of carb-heavy corn and potatoes. Prep time is light if Mock Mashed Potatoes were made earlier in the week. Nutrition information below includes all ingredients in this one dish meal. If your family doesn't like mushrooms, substitute with 1 1/2 cup of chopped broccoli for added nutrition, zero increase in net carbs, and only 6 calories more per serving.

Yield: 6 servings
Serving Size: 10 ounces or 1/6 recipe
Net Carbs per Serving: 4.8 g
Prep Time: 20 minutes
Cook Time: 30 minutes

1 cup onion, chopped
2 cups of mushrooms, thickly sliced
1 tbsp coconut oil
2 pounds ground beef, lean
1 tsp coconut flour
1 tsp salt
1/2 tsp black pepper
1/2 tsp crushed chili pepper flakes
1 cup cheddar cheese, grated
3 cups (approximate) Mock Mashed Potatoes (using riced cauliflower – one complete recipe from Vegetable Dishes)

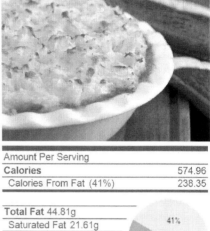

Amount Per Serving	
Calories	574.96
Calories From Fat (41%)	238.35
Total Fat 44.81g	
Saturated Fat 21.61g	
Cholesterol 145.2mg	
Sodium 826.18mg	
Potassium 690.23mg	
Total Carbohydrates 7.87g	
Fiber 3.03g	
Sugar 2.72g	
Protein 34.13g	

KetoHybrid 2014

1. Preheat oven to 350°F.
2. In a large frying pan over medium heat, sauté onion for 5 minutes in coconut oil. Add mushrooms and continue to saute 3 minutes more.
3. Transfer onion and mushrooms to a side bowl.
4. In the same pan, increase heat to medium-high and brown ground beef (5-7 minutes). Add one teaspoon of coconut flour, salt and pepper in the last minute and combine.
5. Transfer meat to a small casserole pan, layer on mushroom and onion mixture, and top with warmed Mock Mashed Potato recipe. Sprinkle with 1/4 cup grated cheese.
6. Bake for 25 to 30 minutes.

Chicken Schnitzel

Think you can't eat breaded and fried foods ever again? This recipe is KetoHybrid approved!

You'll need to have a few items on hand to make this dish – first and foremost, low carb breadcrumbs. Breadcrumbs can be as simple as toasting or drying out any low carb bread that you haven't eaten in time or simply didn't like. You can also grind and add homemade pork rinds, a little coconut or almond flour and some extra Parmesan cheese. Any and all of these items will give you a crispy breading that is safe and reasonable for a low carb high fat menu.

As with any schnitzel recipe, the meat is pounded quite thin, then dredged through beaten egg, coated in crumb, and pan-fried. This recipe is for chicken breast schnitzel but it is also very tasty when made with pork loin pounded thin.

Approximate nutrition information follows. Various crumb options create too wide a range for concise nutritional data.

Yield: 2 servings
Serving Size: One 10" schnitzel or half of yield.
Net Carbs per Serving:: 4 grams
Prep Time: 10 minutes
Cook Time: 30 minutes

2 eggs, lightly beaten
3/4 cup low carb bread crumbs
4 tbsp Parmesan cheese, grated
1/2 tsp salt
1/2 tsp black pepper
1 chicken breast (about 1 pound), cut lengthwise in half
3 tbsp coconut oil
2 tbsp lemon juice (served as wedges but calculated into the recipe)

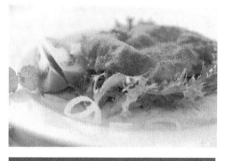

Amount Per Serving	
Calories	571.45
Calories From Fat (52%)	299.33

Total Fat 34.18g	
Saturated Fat 22.29g	
Cholesterol 339.95mg	
Sodium 1101.56mg	
Potassium 952.28mg	
Total Carbohydrates 5.39g	
Fiber 0.38g	
Sugar 0.94g	
Protein 58.98g	

KetoHybrid
2014

1. Beat eggs and transfer to a large plate.

2. Grind crumb, spices, and grated Parmesan cheese and transfer to a second plate.
3. With a meat mallet pound each chicken breast to approximately 1/4" thick.
4. Dip each chicken piece in the beaten egg, and follow by dredging in the crumb mixture.
5. Heat oil in a large non-stick frying pan over medium-low heat.
6. Cook schnitzels individually being careful not to overlap smaller pieces (if any). Brown lightly on both sides (4-5 minutes per side).
7. If serving together, keep warm in a 300°F oven until both schnitzels have finished cooking.
8. Serve with lemon wedges.

Cheese Crusted Wings

These make a great snack as well as the perfect starter to a full meal.

Yield: 20-24 wings
Serving Size: Approximately 5 wings
Net Carbs per Serving: 3.0 grams
Prep Time: 20 minutes
Cook Time: 1 hour

1 pound of chicken wings (about 20-24 wings)
1 1/2 cups Parmesan cheese, grated
1 tsp parsley flakes
2 tsp garlic powder
1 tsp white pepper
1/2 cup butter, melted

1. Preheat oven to 350°F. Lightly oil a non-stick baking dish.
2. In a large bowl combine cheese and spices.
3. Dip each wing first in melted butter and then in the cheese mixture.
4. Bake uncovered for 1 hour.

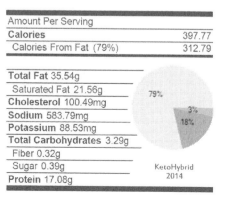

Amount Per Serving	
Calories	397.77
Calories From Fat (79%)	312.79
Total Fat 35.54g	
Saturated Fat 21.56g	
Cholesterol 100.49mg	
Sodium 583.79mg	
Potassium 88.53mg	
Total Carbohydrates 3.29g	
Fiber 0.32g	
Sugar 0.39g	
Protein 17.08g	

KetoHybrid
2014

Tamatar Murghi – Indian Chicken

An easy complete meal. Exudes a taste of India, sure to impress your guests. Spicy and flavorful without intense heat. You can just as easily cook it on the stove top, but I like to put it all in a crockpot and let the aroma fill the kitchen.

Yield: 4 servings

Serving Size: 1/4 finished recipe, approximately 2 cups

Net Carbs per Serving: 9.2 grams

Prep Time: 10-15 minutes

Cook Time: 45 minutes

3 cups cauliflower florets (1 medium sized cauliflower)

2 pounds chicken breast, boneless, skinless

3 tbsp olive or coconut oil

2 tbsp butter

1/2 tsp salt

1/2 tsp white pepper

1/2 cup onion, chopped

1/2 tsp garlic powder

1/2 tsp turmeric

1 tbsp ginger, ground

1 1/2 cups home made chicken stock

1 tbsp tomato paste

1 cup heavy cream

Amount Per Serving	
Calories	669.03
Calories From Fat (59%)	397.71
Total Fat 45.23g	
Saturated Fat 27.83g	
Cholesterol 244.63mg	
Sodium 761.95mg	
Potassium 1292.55mg	
Total Carbohydrates 12.04g	
Fiber 2.19g	
Sugar 4.32g	
Protein 53.63g	

59%

7%

34%

KetoHybrid
2014

1. Parboil or steam cauliflower in a small amount of water for about 5 minutes; drain.
2. Cut each chicken breast in bite-size pieces.
3. To a 6 quart crock pot, add 3 tbsp oil and 2 tbsp butter.
4. Add chicken pieces and sprinkle with salt and pepper.
5. Add finely chopped onion and sprinkle with spices.
6. Add broth and tomato paste.
7. Add cauliflower.
8. Cook on low setting for 4 hours or high for 2 hours.
9. Ten minutes before serving, stir in cream, replace the lid and turn off the crock pot.

Parmesan Encrusted Chicken Fingers

Pub food that's better for you! Every week we cook more than we need, then slice and eat cold in a salad for lunch or dinners when we're short on time.

Serving Size: 4 ounces or 1/4 entire recipe
Net Carb per serving: 0.6 gram
Prep Time: 20 minutes
Cook Time: 1 hour

1 pound chicken breast, boneless, skinless (approximately 2 small breasts)
1/2 tsp salt
1 tsp white pepper
1/2 cup Parmesan cheese, grated
4 tbsp mayonnaise

1. Preheat oven to 425°F.
2. Place mayonnaise on one small plate; Parmesan cheese with salt and pepper, on another.
3. Cut chicken breasts into similar sized fingers.
4. Roll each chicken finger first in mayonnaise, then in cheese, and set on a small baking sheet or casserole. These should be uncrowded and evenly spaced.
5. Bake for 25 minutes.

Amount Per Serving	
Calories	287.24
Calories From Fat (56%)	160.98

Total Fat 18.19g	56%
Saturated Fat 4.43g	
Cholesterol 83.58mg	1%
Sodium 686.27mg	
Potassium 437.58mg	43%
Total Carbohydrates 0.76g	
Fiber 0.08g	
Sugar 0.16g	KetoHybrid
Protein 28.91g	2014

Moroccan Chicken Tagine

The word tagine is used both for the richly spiced Moroccan stew as it is the traditional pot it is cooked in. Your slow cooker will do the same work as a tagine although you may not feel as 'authentic'.

Tagine recipes often have sweet potatoes, carrots, chickpeas, apricots and raisins added in. To keep our meals low carb, we pair the recipe below with summer squash (grilled zucchini or yellow crookneck squash) and cauliflower.

This is the perfect stew for a cool, rainy day. A lovely indulgence when you need a break from typical North American flavors: cream, cheese, garlic and thyme. This tagine's spice blend is heady, warming, and almost sweet.

Make this recipe your own favorite by converting it to pork, fish or beef – allow denser meats a longer marinate and cook time. Try the recipe first with chicken though, it will be hard not to fall in love with it.

Net Carbs per Serving: 5.1 g

Serves: 4

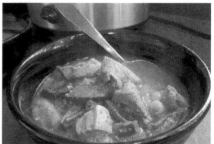

2 tbsp olive oil

1/2 cup onion, diced

1 tbsp garlic, minced

2 cups homemade chicken stock

1/4 tsp saffron (optional, but lovely)

1 tsp black pepper

1 tsp cumin

1 tsp cinnamon

1 1/2 pounds chicken breast (about 2 medium to large sized breasts)

1/4 cup almonds

2 tbsp green olives, chopped

1 tbsp tomato paste

1 tsp lime juice

1/2 tsp lime zest

Garnish: 2 tbsp cilantro, fresh chopped

1. In a small frying pan over medium high heat, saute onion and garlic in 2 tablespoons olive oil.

2. To crock pot add homemade chicken stock and spices. Turn to high heat, allowing the stock to warm while preparing other ingredients.
3. Chop chicken breast into 1" pieces and once the stock has warmed to room temperature or above, add chicken to the stock with remaining ingredients.
4. Turn the crock pot to low, cover and cook for 2 hours.
5. To serve, spoon equal portions of tagine into large soup bowls and garnish with a teaspoon or more of freshly chopped cilantro.

Amount Per Serving	
Calories	350.43
Calories From Fat (42%)	148.52

Total Fat 16.93g	
Saturated Fat 2.52g	42%
Cholesterol 108.86mg	
Sodium 639.13mg	8%
Potassium 910.89mg	50%
Total Carbohydrates 7.51g	
Fiber 2.4g	
Sugar 2.12g	KetoHybrid
Protein 41.26g	2014

Cheesy Broccoli Chicken

Another one-dish chicken dinner that can be made ahead and re-heated or served right from the crock pot. When on a budget, we've also made this with cheddar cheese.

Yield: Dinner for 6
Serving Size: 2 cups that include 1/2 pound chicken
Net Carbs per Serving: 7 grams
Prep Time: 20 minutes
Cook Time: 30 minutes

3 pounds chicken breast, boneless, skinless, cut into 6 equal portions
2 cups broccoli, cut into florets (about 1 1/2 bunches)
4 tbsp butter
3 tbsp olive oil
1 pound button mushrooms, sliced (20-22 medium)
1 tbsp coconut flour
1 tbsp lemon juice
1/2 cup chicken stock
1/2 cup dry white wine (a cooking wine is fine)
1 1/2 cups Swiss cheese, grated
1/2 tsp salt
1 tsp black pepper
1/2 cup Swiss cheese, grated for top

1. Steam broccoli until slightly tender, 3-5 minutes and place in a lightly oiled, large casserole dish.
2. In three tablespoons of olive oil over medium heat, cook chicken until juices run clear – about 3-5 minutes on each side. Layer the chicken pieces over the broccoli, squeezing approximately 1 tablespoon of lemon juice evenly over the chicken.
3. Preheat broiler to high setting.
4. Melt 3 tablespoons of butter in the pan you used to cook the chicken and cook mushrooms over medium-high heat until tender – about 3 to 5 minutes.
5. Turn heat to low and remove mushroom slices from the pan with a slotted spoon, leaving liquid in the pan.
6. To the pan, add remaining 2 tablespoons of butter and whisk in coconut flour. Continue to cook, stirring for 3 minutes more.

7. Add chicken stock and wine to the pan and continue to whisk until blended and sauce begins to thicken slightly. Add 1 1/2 cups of shredded Swiss cheese, salt and pepper, and stir until completely melted.
8. Pour the contents of the pan over the chicken and broccoli. Top with cooked mushroom slices and the last 1/2 cup of grated cheese.
9. Place the casserole pan on the top rack of your oven (5-6 inches from the top) and broil until the cheese on top begins to bubble – 5-6 minutes.
10. Refrigerate leftovers. Reheat in a 350°F oven for 20 minutes.

Amount Per Serving	
Calories	533.03
Calories From Fat (32%)	172.35
Total Fat 25.8g	
Saturated Fat 13.72g	
Cholesterol 202.01mg	
Sodium 565.54mg	
Potassium 1265.85mg	
Total Carbohydrates 9.25g	
Fiber 2.13g	
Sugar 2.57g	
Protein 61.73g	

32%
26%
1%
40%

KetoHybrid
2014

Rosemary Leg of Lamb

For celebration or Sunday dinners with the family. This traditionally easy and impressive entree is best when using fresh herbs (but still compares well using dried herbs).

Yield: 6 servings
Serving Size: 4-6 ounces cooked lamb
Net Carbs per Serving: 2.5 g
Prep Time: 8 hours to marinate, 20 minutes of prep
Cook Time: 90 minutes

3 pounds boneless leg of lamb
2 tbsp rosemary
1 tbsp thyme
3 tbsp garlic, minced
1 tbsp mustard, Dijon style
1 tsp salt
3/4 tsp black pepper
6 tbsp olive oil
1/4 cup dry red wine
1 tsp balsamic vinegar
1 tsp mustard, Dijon style
1/2 tsp salt
1/2 tsp pepper

Amount Per Serving	
Calories	599.27
Calories From Fat (66%)	398.35

Total Fat 44.47g	
Saturated Fat 15.12g	66%
Cholesterol 151.96mg	
Sodium 754.7mg	
Potassium 648.3mg	30%
Total Carbohydrates 3.34g	
Fiber 0.86g	
Sugar 0.12g	KetoHybrid
Protein 42.76g	2014

1. Make an herb rub of rosemary, thyme, garlic, mustard, salt, and pepper in a food processor or mortar and pestle. Mix with 6 tablespoons of olive oil to create a paste.
2. Rub paste on all sides of lamb leg, concentrating mostly on the thicker end. Cover and refrigerate in a shallow glass baking dish for 8 hours or longer.
3. Preheat oven to 425°F and roast the lamb leg for 10 minutes. Reduce heat to 350°F for 1 1/2 hours. Once cooked, remove lamb from the baking dish, cover, and allow to rest 10 minutes before carving from the bone.
4. While lamb leg is resting, make your sauce in a small pan over medium-low heat by combining pan juices, red wine, balsamic vinegar, and mustard.
5. Add salt and pepper to taste (approximately 1/2 teaspoon of each). Serve alongside the lamb.

Tuna Patties

The perfect low carb base for a tuna melt sandwich on one of our English Muffins. Also makes a delicious crunchy addition to a dinner salad. Try them once; even if you don't like tuna; they may become one of your new favorites.

Yield: 4 patties
Serving Size: 2 patties
Net Carbs per Serving: 4.1 grams
Prep Time: 10 minutes
Cook Time: 5-8 minutes

6 ounce can tuna, packed in water
1/4 cup scallions, minced (about 2, both green and white sections)
2 tbsp parsley flakes (or fresh)
1/2 tsp salt
1/4 tsp thyme
1/8 tsp white pepper
4 ounces chopped walnuts
2 eggs, slightly beaten
2 tbsp coconut oil

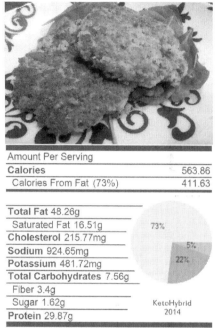

Amount Per Serving	
Calories	563.86
Calories From Fat (73%)	411.63

Total Fat 48.26g	
Saturated Fat 16.51g	73%
Cholesterol 215.77mg	
Sodium 924.65mg	5%
Potassium 481.72mg	22%
Total Carbohydrates 7.56g	
Fiber 3.4g	
Sugar 1.62g	KetoHybrid
Protein 29.87g	2014

1. In a small bowl, combine drained tuna, scallions, parsley, salt, white pepper, thyme, chopped walnuts, and beaten eggs.
2. Warm coconut oil in a large non-stick frying pan over medium heat.
3. Create 4 equal sized patties by spooning tuna mixture into the four quadrants of the pan. Flatten slightly if required.
4. Cook on both sides – about 3-4 minutes per side.
5. Serve immediately or cool on a wire rack for 10 minutes before refrigerating.

Teriyaki Glazed Salmon

Traditionally teriyaki sauce is high in sugar and would be off the menu for KetoHybrid dieters. We've come up with a low carb solution; made possibly by a marinade and ample time. Same great flavor, far fewer carbohydrates. Apply this same concept to either pork or chicken.

If you have a brown sugar substitute on hand, use it instead of real sugar and you can decrease net carbs considerably.

Serves: 6
Net Carbs per Serving: 5.1 g (or 3.3 if using sugar substitute)
Prep Time: 10 minutes (plus 1 hour minimum marinade)
Cook Time: 15 minutes

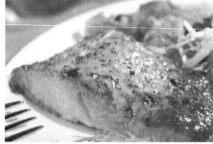

1 1/2 pounds salmon, fresh
1/2 cup low-sodium soy sauce
2 tbsp white vinegar
1 tbsp fresh garlic, minced
1 tbsp ground ginger
3/4 tbsp brown sugar
1/2 cup green onions, finely chopped
(both white and green sections)

1. Divide salmon into 6 equal portions.
2. In a glass baking dish, combine all ingredients except salmon and mix well.
3. Add salmon – ensuring that each piece is amply covered by the marinade.
4. Refrigerate for 1-8 hours.
5. Preheat oven to 350°F and bake salmon with marinade for 10-15 minutes or until the fish flakes easily with a fork.

Amount Per Serving	
Calories	170.6
Calories From Fat (27%)	45.55

Total Fat 5.06g	
Saturated Fat 0.95g	
Cholesterol 52.13mg	
Sodium 795.66mg	
Potassium 501.79mg	
Total Carbohydrates 5.6g	
Fiber 0.55g	
Sugar 2.27g	
Protein 24.68g	

27%
12%
61%

KetoHybrid
2014

Salmon Steaks & Chive Butter

Serves: 4
Net Carbs per Serving: 0.06 grams
Prep Time: 5 minutes
Cook Time: 15 minutes

6 salmon steaks (4 ounces each, about 1" thick)
1 tbsp olive oil

Chive Butter:
10 tbsp butter, softened
2 tsp parsley, minced
2 tbsp fresh chives, minced

1. Blend parsley and chives into soft butter. Refrigerate until hardened.
2. Brush salmon with olive oil, and grill on medium-high, 5-6 minutes per side.
3. Transfer salmon to individual plates, then top with a large pat of chilled chive butter.

Amount Per Serving	
Calories	500.83
Calories From Fat (70%)	350.46

Total Fat 39.66g	
Saturated Fat 20.08g	70%
Cholesterol 154.52mg	
Sodium 131.69mg	0%
Potassium 636.94mg	30%
Total Carbohydrates 0.11g	
Fiber 0.05g	
Sugar 0.05g	KetoHybrid
Protein 35.21g	2014

Making Bacon

Delicious nitrate free bacon with a process you control from start to finish. Superior in flavor to a grocery store bacon; generally cheaper overall, and free of chemicals, over-salting, and added sugars. (If you don't think there are added sugars in bacon from the grocery store – check the label, you'll see the additives and the elevated carbohydrate count.)

This is my favorite bacon recipe but you can adjust spices, herbs, and garlic to your taste (leave the salt at 2 tbsp per 2 pounds of pork belly though).

2 lbs pork belly, skin on
2 tbsp unrefined sea salt
1 tbsp freshly ground black pepper
1 tsp rosemary (dried or 2 tsp fresh minced)
1 tsp dried thyme
1 tsp dried fennel seed
2 bay leaves
1 garlic clove, minced

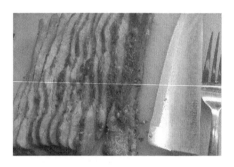

1. Place the pork belly in a large colander and run under cold water. Allow to dry for 2 minutes.
2. Combine all seasonings in a food grade plastic bag large enough to hold the pork belly. I find the large freezer bags work perfectly.
3. Add the pork belly to your spice bag and shake well to cover the pork belly with spices.
4. Refrigerate for one week, shaking the bag daily.
5. At 7-10 days, remove the pork belly from the bag and rinse well under cold water.
6. Roast the pork belly on a baking sheet for 2 hours at 200°F. Internal meat temperature should read 150°F.
7. Allow the bacon to cool, then transfer to a cutting board. Slice off and discard the skin. If you're making pork rinds, try to keep the fat attached to the skin at a minimum.
8. Slice the bacon into thin strips, or leave whole to slice as needed. Refrigerate in a new food grade plastic bag.

Pork Rinds

Pork rinds (aka crackling or crackle) are roasted or deep fried pork skin. Although it may sound odd, they are enjoyed in many cultures as a snack or dipper.

Local butchers are happy to sell pork skin (usually cheaper than the cost of soup bones), but you may need to give them a few days notice to save some for you. Far better is to buy pork bellies, skin on, to make bacon. Once cured, you can use that skin to make rinds.

We keep our weekly supply in the refrigerator and grind them up to replace or supplement breadcrumbs.

You'll need:
a very sharp knife
roasting pan with a wire rack insert
pork skin
unrefined sea salt

1. If you are using the skin from your cured bacon skip to step #4.
2. Wash then cut the skin into strips, approximately 1-2" wide by 3" long.
3. Place strips on a baking sheet or plate, fat side down. Dust with salt.
4. The next day, flip strips (fat side up) and dust again with salt. Return to the fridge for 24 hours more.
5. Preheat oven to 400°F.
6. Add 1/2 inch of water to bottom of roasting pan, then set the rinds on the rack, fat side down. The water catches the fat as it runs off the rinds, ensuring that they don't burn or cook in their own hot fat.
7. Bake for 20 minutes, then turn the oven down to 300°F. Bake for another hour.
8. Turn oven up to 350°F and continue baking for another 20 minutes.
9. Remove from the oven and allow to cool before handling. Refrigerate up to 7 days, or grind and keep in the freezer to use as a breadcrumb replacement.

Slow Cooked Pulled Pork

A spicy 'pulled' meat dish traditionally made with beef but you can substitute with turkey or pork and have it be just as delicious!

Serves: 12

Prep Time: 10 minutes

Cook Time: 6 hours

Net Carbs per Serving: 4.4 g

4 lbs pork roast (butt or shoulder)

1/2 cup water

Pulled Pork Sauce:

1 tbsp olive oil

3 cups tomatoes, fresh, diced

2 tbsp red onion, finely chopped

1 tbsp garlic, minced

1 small can tomato paste (6 ounces)

2 tbsp white vinegar

1 tablespoon Worcestershire sauce

1 tsp chili pepper flakes

1 tsp cumin, ground

1/2 tsp oregano

1/2 tsp coriander leaves, dried

1 tbsp liquid smoke (optional but delicious)

1 tbsp salt

1 tsp black pepper

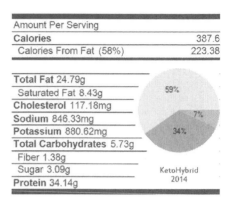

Amount Per Serving	
Calories	387.6
Calories From Fat (58%)	223.38

Total Fat 24.79g	
Saturated Fat 8.43g	
Cholesterol 117.18mg	
Sodium 846.33mg	
Potassium 880.62mg	
Total Carbohydrates 5.73g	
Fiber 1.38g	
Sugar 3.09g	
Protein 34.14g	

KetoHybrid
2014

1. Add all sauce ingredients to a food processor and puree.
2. Add water, pork roast and 1/2 pulled pork sauce to a 4 quart crock pot and cook on high for 6 hours.
3. Thirty minutes before serving, remove the meat to a cutting board. Leave the slow cooker on low with the lid off.
4. Slice the meat across the grain into 3-4" pieces. Next, pull at and shred the meat using both hands, a fork in each hand.
5. Return meat to the slow cooker with remaining sauce and cook for a further 20 minutes on low (lid off if sauce is too thin; lid on it sauce is a perfect consistency).

Scotch Eggs

Deep fried balls of delicious! A spicy sausage patty encases a soft boiled egg – traditionally eaten on Christmas eve or at cocktail parties. These are time consuming to make, but worth the effort. I usually make a double batch; within 24 hours they have all disappeared!*

This is the only item I deep fry and I do so in the lard on hand from making bacon. Frying in lard isn't quirky, it is considered by many experts to be the healthiest way to fry foods. Scotch Eggs can also be baked – 375°F for 30 minutes or until done – but I can never get the sausage to stay on the egg.

Yield: 6 servings
Serving Size: 1 Scotch Egg
Net Carbs per Serving: 0.9 grams
Prep Time: 30 minutes
Cook Time: 10-50 minutes

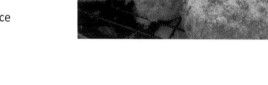

6 eggs, soft boiled and peeled
1 pound ground pork
2 tsp Worcestershire sauce
2 tsp Dijon mustard
1/4 teaspoon cumin
1/4 teaspoon oregano
1/4 teaspoon cayenne
1 egg, beaten
1/2 cup low carb breadcrumbs (mixed with finely ground pork rinds or parmesan cheese)

1. Mix Worchestershire, Dijon, cumin, oregano, and cayenne pepper into ground pork.
2. Divide ground pork into 6 equal portions and wrap each portion around each egg.
3. Roll each scotch egg into the raw beaten egg, and then roll in the bread crumb mixture.
4. Deep fry until golden brown – about 10 minutes. Keep cooked Scotch Eggs warm in a 350°F oven until all have been cooked.

*If you are making a large batch of these, refrigerate each egg after encasing in sausage until ready to cook.

This nutritional information is an estimate only. You must increase nutrition data by 10-15% in both fats and calories due to deep frying.

Amount Per Serving	
Calories	330.86
Calories From Fat (66%)	218.76

Total Fat 24.28g	
Saturated Fat 8.73g	66%
Cholesterol 279.35mg	1%
Sodium 314.05mg	
Potassium 327.42mg	33%
Total Carbohydrates 0.98g	
Fiber 0.1g	
Sugar 0.4g	KetoHybrid
Protein 25.3g	2014

CHAPTER 21

Vegetable Entrees and Side Dishes

The easiest way to love the KetoHybrid diet is to learn a variety of ways to enjoy non-starchy, high sugar vegetables.

Make friends with every green vegetable, even if that means loading on the butter, garlic infused olive oil, coconut oil, and cheeses (you need those fats in your diet anyway). I'd also urge you to try roasting or grilling every vegetable in your grocery store, at least once. The flavors that are hidden in vegetables until they've been roasted – superb. Remember those over-boiled, watery Brussels sprouts your mom forced you to eat? They're a crunchy, almost sweet treat when roasted!

Every week our grocery list includes a few heads of cauliflower and a big bag of zucchini. Both are incredibly versatile once you learn a few tricks and get to know the spices in your cupboard.

Zucchini is easily spiraled with an inexpensive device[16] to look like spaghetti noodles that cook up in 3 minutes (above). As long as you have a strong flavored sauce, you're not likely to notice that you're eating an incredibly healthy meal; and it cooks faster than pasta.

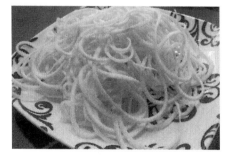

---

16 www.KetoHybrid.com/spiralizer

Cauliflower dices, mashes, and rices. With a creamy cheese sauce it mimics the traditional Macaroni and Cheese dish, can mash into a sturdy crust for pizza, and easily fakes a risotto when riced.

Finally, be sure to have a look through the vegetable list in the carbohydrate counts section of this book. It will help to familiarize you with options for healthy eating and you may be surprised by a few naturally healthy foods, that are actually quite high in carbs.

Oven-Roasted Brussels Sprouts

Yield: 4 cups

Serving Size: 1 cup

Net Carbs per Serving: 5.4 grams

Prep Time: 10 minutes

Cook Time: 20 minutes

4 cups Brussels sprouts (about 1 pound)

1 1/2 tablespoons olive oil

1 tbsp garlic, minced

1/2 tsp salt

1/4 tsp black pepper

Amount Per Serving	
Calories	86.83
Calories From Fat (54%)	47.12

Total Fat 5.34g	
Saturated Fat 0.76g	
Cholesterol 0mg	
Sodium 313.26mg	
Potassium 354.7mg	
Total Carbohydrates 8.83g	
Fiber 3.43g	
Sugar 1.96g	
Protein 3.15g	

54%
9%
37%

KetoHybrid
2014

1. Preheat oven to 425°F.
2. Slice washed and trimmed Brussels sprouts in half lengthwise and place in a large bowl.
3. Add remaining ingredients to the bowl and toss.
4. Bake Brussels sprouts on a baking sheet for 15-20 minutes on the middle rack. Stir the sprouts once during roasting time.
5. Remove them from the oven when they are slightly seared and crispy on the outside, juicy and tender on the inside.

Fast Lemon Garlic Broccoli

From frozen to fabulous in 20 minutes. While we're not huge fans of frozen vegetables, they are helpful for cooks with busy lives.

Yield: 4 servings

Serving Size: 1 cup

Net Carbs per Serving: 4.7 grams

Prep Time: 12 minutes

Cook Time: 10 minutes

4 cups broccoli spears, frozen

2 1/2 tbsp butter

2 tsp garlic, minced

2 tsp lemon zest

1/2 tsp salt

1/3 tsp black pepper

Amount Per Serving	
Calories	118.15
Calories From Fat (55%)	65.14
Total Fat 7.42g	
Saturated Fat 4.6g	
Cholesterol 19.08mg	
Sodium 770.39mg	
Potassium 342.93mg	
Total Carbohydrates 10.58g	
Fiber 5.7g	
Sugar 2.71g	
Protein 5.9g	

55%
13% 32%

KetoHybrid
2014

1. Melt butter in a large frying pan over medium heat and lightly saute minced garlic for 1-2 minutes.
2. Stir broccoli into the pan, and continue to cook for 7-8 minutes.
3. Stir in lemon zest, salt, and pepper. Serve immediately.

Roasted Asparagus

Asparagus is readily available and relatively inexpensive, year round. It is also a great vehicle for added fats when you need to adjust your meal's fat content – its as simple as topping with extra butter or as decadent as whipping up a bit of Hollandaise sauce (you'll find an easy recipe in the Sauces section). This recipe also converts well for the outdoor grill.

Yield: About 20 spears

Serving Size: 1/4 recipe, 4-5 spears each

Net Carbs per Serving: 2.6 grams

Prep Time: 5 minutes

Cook Time: 10-15 minutes

1 pound asparagus spears (15-20 stalks)

Amount Per Serving	
Calories	84.77
Calories From Fat (72%)	60.89
Total Fat 6.9g	
Saturated Fat 0.98g	
Cholesterol 0mg	
Sodium 148.01mg	
Potassium 236.52mg	
Total Carbohydrates 4.95g	
Fiber 2.44g	
Sugar 2.15g	
Protein 2.6g	

72%
21%
7%

KetoHybrid
2014

2 tbsp olive oil

2 tsp garlic, minced

1/4 teaspoon salt

1/4 teaspoon black pepper

1. Preheat oven to 400°F.
2. Wash, and trim asparagus (remove approximately 1" of the woody bottom). Place spears on a small baking sheet.
3. Mix remaining ingredients in a small bowl and drizzle over the asparagus.
4. Roast on the middle rack for 10-12 minutes or until slightly tender. Thicker stalks need extra cooking time.

Smokey Almond Beans

A delicious and quick way to serve beans fresh from the Farmer's Market. The recipe is simple but the impact of a few extra ingredients is delightful.

Yield: 3 cups

Serving Size: 1/2 cup

Net Carbs per Serving: 3.6 grams

Prep Time: 15 to 20 minutes

Cook Time: 12 to 15 minutes

3 cups fresh beans, washed and trimmed (approximately 1 pound)

1 1/2 tbsp olive oil

1 tsp garlic, crushed

1/2 cup almonds, coarsely chopped

1/2 tsp chipotle pepper, finely chopped

Amount Per Serving	
Calories	95.08
Calories From Fat (67%)	63.64
Total Fat 7.42g	
Saturated Fat 0.79g	
Cholesterol 0mg	
Sodium 3.75mg	
Potassium 179.5mg	
Total Carbohydrates 6.14g	
Fiber 2.49g	
Sugar 2.13g	
Protein 2.8g	

67%

24%

9%

KetoHybrid 2014

1. In a small sauce pan, with just enough water, boil trimmed beans with coarsely chopped pepper for 10 minutes, or until nearly cooked. Drain in a colander.
2. Lightly saute garlic in oil, in a large frying pan over medium heat for 1-2 minutes. Stir in chopped almonds and cook one minute more.
3. Add drained beans with the pepper to the pan. Lightly sauteing 2 minutes more.
4. Serve immediately. Easily reheats for meals later in the week.

Faux Mac and Cheese

Soon to be your favorite way to enjoy a classic dish! The trick into having this dish feel more like a traditional mac 'n cheese, is in the firmness and cut of the cauliflower.

Store any leftovers in the refrigerator up to one week. Reheats nicely in a microwave or covered dish in a warmed oven.

Yield: 3 cups

Serving Size: 1/2 cup, 1/6 recipe, or 4 1/2 ounces

Net Carbs per Serving: 4 grams

Prep Time: 15 minutes

Cook Time: 20 minutes

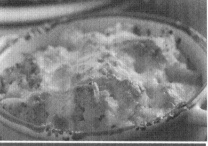

Amount Per Serving	
Calories	253.86
Calories From Fat (73%)	184.78

Total Fat 21.03g	
Saturated Fat 12.88g	
Cholesterol 66.34mg	
Sodium 424.62mg	
Potassium 248.33mg	
Total Carbohydrates 5.07g	
Fiber 1.08g	
Sugar 1.66g	
Protein 12.17g	

KetoHybrid 2014

3 cups cauliflower, cut into small florets (1 small head)

3/4 cup heavy cream

3 ounces cream cheese

2 teaspoons Dijon mustard

8 ounces sharp Cheddar cheese, shredded (2 cups)

1/8 teaspoon garlic powder

1/4 teaspoon salt

1/4 teaspoon black pepper

1. Preheat oven to 375°F.
2. Cook cauliflower in boiling water about 5 minutes or until slightly done. Allow to drain well.
3. In a small saucepan over medium heat, warm the cream, then whisk in cream cheese and mustard. Add 1 1/2 cups of cheddar and spices and continue gently whisking for 1-2 minutes more or fully melted and a consistent sauce has been made.
4. Place cauliflower in a baking dish, add warmed cheese sauce and gently stir to combine. Top with remaining cheddar and bake until the top has browned, about 15 minutes.

Mock Mashed Potatoes

Do you have a favorite recipe that calls for mashed potatoes but now feel that you can't enjoy it ever again? Fret not! These creamy mock mashed potatoes work as well as a side dish as they do crowning your favorite Shepherd's Pie recipe.

Yield: 1 1/2 cups

Serving Size: 1/2 cup

Net Carbs per Serving: 3.4 grams

Prep Time: 15 minutes

Cook Time: 40 minutes

3 cups cauliflower, cut into small florets (about 1 head)

2 tbsp cream

2 tbsp butter, melted

1/2 tsp salt

1/8 tsp white pepper

Amount Per Serving	
Calories	106.17
Calories From Fat (75%)	79.97

Total Fat 9.11g		
Saturated Fat 5.64g	75%	
Cholesterol 24.05mg		
Sodium 422.73mg	19%	
Potassium 314.43mg	6%	
Total Carbohydrates 5.47g		
Fiber 2.03g		
Sugar 1.93g	KetoHybrid	
Protein 2.31g	2014	

1. Steam cauliflower until quite soft (10 minutes).
2. Allow cauliflower to cool, then puree with remaining ingredients in a blender or food processor.
3. Serve immediately as a side, use in other recipes in place of mashed potatoes, or store in the refrigerator up to one week.

Faux Hash Browns

A delicious low carb addition to your breakfast. Two small hash brown patties at less than 2 net carbs.

Yield: 8 hash browns

Serving Size: 2 pieces

Net Carbs per Serving: 1.8 grams

Prep Time: 15 minutes

Cook Time: 5 minutes

1 egg

1 teaspoon paprika

1/2 tsp salt

1/4 tsp black pepper

1/4 tsp garlic powder

2 slices cooked bacon, chopped (about 3 tbsp, 1/6 pound)

2 tbsp onion, finely chopped

1 1/2 cups cooked cauliflower, grated

2 tbsp coconut oil, for frying

Amount Per Serving	
Calories	114.47
Calories From Fat (77%)	87.93
Total Fat 9.9g	
Saturated Fat 1.92g	
Cholesterol 50.9mg	
Sodium 408.68mg	
Potassium 130.47mg	
Total Carbohydrates 3.06g	
Fiber 1.41g	
Sugar 1.29g	
Protein 4.09g	

77%

9%

14%

KetoHybrid
2014

1. Mix all ingredients except cauliflower and oil in a medium sized bowl.
2. Fold in grated cauliflower and stir just until mixed.
3. In a large skillet, warm 1/2 the oil over medium high heat. For every hash brown, drop 1/8 of the mixture (approximately one heaping tablespoon) into the pan and slightly flatten. Cook for 2 minutes on each side until golden brown.
4. Serve immediately.

Leafy Mediterranean Salad

I'd never try a diet that didn't include this salad. This version had to go easy on the tomato, to keep carb counts low. Some days, I toss everything together in one bowl – dinner for one!

Yield: 2 side salads
Serving Size: 1/2 recipe, about 4 cups
Net Carbs per Serving: 6.6
Prep Time: 10 minutes

3 cups mixed salad greens
1/4 cup sweet red pepper, diced
1/4 cup fresh tomato, chopped
(preferably plum tomato)
1 cup cucumber, chopped
1/4 cup red or purple onion, sliced thin
4 ounces Feta cheese, cubed or crumbled
12 whole black olives, pit removed

Dressing:
1/2 tsp garlic, minced
1 tbsp olive oil
1/2 tsp balsamic vinegar
2 tsp basil, fresh and chopped
1/4 tsp black pepper

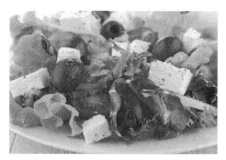

Amount Per Serving	
Calories	277.51
Calories From Fat (69%)	192.54

Total Fat 21.94g	
Saturated Fat 9.8g	69%
Cholesterol 50.46mg	
Sodium 874.87mg	15%
Potassium 363.49mg	15%
Total Carbohydrates 11.25g	
Fiber 3.54g	
Sugar 4.82g	KetoHybrid
Protein 10.16g	2014

1. Mix dressing ingredients in a small bowl.
2. Divide salad greens between 2 salad plates.
3. Top greens with remaining ingredients, drizzle on the dressing, and enjoy.

Coleslaw

Yield: 4 cups
Serving Size: 1/2 cup
Net Carbs per Serving: 2.6 grams
Prep Time: 15 minutes
Time to Table: 6-8 hours

4 cups cabbage, finely shredded
(medium cabbage, about 7"
diameter)
1/2 cup grated carrot
3/4 cup KetoHybrid mayonnaise
(recipe in Sauces section)
3 tbsp white vinegar
1 tsp garlic, minced
1⁄2 tsp celery seed
1/4 tsp white pepper
1⁄2 tsp salt

Amount Per Serving	
Calories	142.49
Calories From Fat (88%)	125.24
Total Fat 14.16g	
Saturated Fat 2.08g	
Cholesterol 22.51mg	
Sodium 308.95mg	
Potassium 110.94mg	
Total Carbohydrates 3.98g	
Fiber 1.36g	
Sugar 1.78g	
Protein 1.03g	

88%
10%
2%

KetoHybrid
2014

1. In a large bowl, mix the mayonnaise, vinegar and and spices.
2. Add the shredded cabbage and carrot and toss to coat.
3. Cover and refrigerate 6-8 hours for best results.

Zucchini and Feta Fritters – Kolokithokeftedes

From Greece comes a delicious appetizer named Kolokithokeftedes. This is traditionally served with tsatziki, sour cream or applesauce. They are made as a flat fritter or formed into round balls; usually fried, but occasionally baked.

The texture of a fried food mixed with the saltiness of feta and those Mediterranean spices will have you feeling like you're cheating. At less than 1 net carb per fritter you can eat these a different way every day. Pop a poached egg on one for breakfast. Fry them up thin and firm for the 'bread' of your open-face tuna salad sandwich. Cut each one into 4 – 1" wide strips and add them to your lunch plate of finger foods. The possibilities are endless.

The ingredients in this recipe are relatively inexpensive so I urge to you experiment. Zucchini pairs well with many spices – both sweet and savory. Try swapping out the basil/oregano combo for a chipotle/red pepper mix and use cheddar instead of feta. Or keep the basil but substitute the feta with freshly grated parmesan. Finally, if you're craving something sweet, replace the spices/scallions/cheese for a cinnamon/nutmeg/applesauce variation (recipe below).

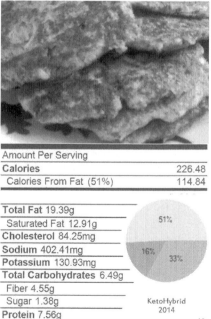

Yield: 12 fritters
Serving Size: 2 fritters
Net Carbs per Serving: 2.0 grams
Prep Time: 15 minutes
Cook Time: 10-30 minutes

2 cups grated zucchini
1/4 tsp salt
1/4 cup flax seed, ground
2 tbsp coconut flour
2 tsp basil, dried
1 tsp oregano, dried
1 cup crumbled feta
1/4 cup scallions, chopped
2 large eggs
4 tbsp coconut oil or butter, for frying

Amount Per Serving	
Calories	226.48
Calories From Fat (51%)	114.84

Total Fat 19.39g	
Saturated Fat 12.91g	
Cholesterol 84.25mg	
Sodium 402.41mg	
Potassium 130.93mg	
Total Carbohydrates 6.49g	
Fiber 4.55g	
Sugar 1.38g	
Protein 7.56g	

KetoHybrid
2014

1. Grate zucchini, wrap in a clean kitchen towel and wring out all moisture.
2. In a large bowl, combine flax seed meal, coconut flour, oregano, basil, and salt. Stir in feta and scallions, zucchini and eggs. Mix until thoroughly combined.
3. Form mixture into 12 patties 3-4 inches in diameter, 3/4" thick.
4. In a large skillet, over medium high heat, melt half of the coconut oil or butter until hot enough to saute.
5. Cook as many fritters as will fit in the pan until crispy and brown on both sides; 3-4 minutes per side.
6. Remove to wire rack while cooking the remaining fritters.
7. Serve warm or refrigerate up to 1 week.

CHAPTER 22

All The Little Extras

Mayonnaise

You're going to eat mayonnaise, let's make sure it is the healthiest version possible. KetoHybrid, organic, paleo, low carb, or just counting calories – whatever the diet, the five minutes it takes to whip up a batch of mayonnaise will be time well spent.

Mayonnaise is in quite a few of this book's recipes which is why I'm such a stickler about exposing the contents of this grocery store staple.

Start by comparing the mayo in your fridge to the recipe below. You'll find the first ingredient listed is either canola or soybean oil (likely GMO oils), even though the colorful label on the front states olive oil (usually only trace amounts are in the contents). You'll also find added sugar and more than a few ingredients you may not recognize. All red flags. A creamy, savory, and simple-to-make condiment has no need for oils of questionable quality, sugar, or chemicals.

Plus the average store mayo has 100 calories per tablespoon and contains 90mg sodium.

KetoHybrid Mayo has 13% fewer calories, 1/2 the sodium, 30% fewer ingredients, no artificial acids or chemicals, and zero added sugar. It also tastes better.

As with all homemade condiments, your biggest challenge will be getting the oils to emulsify (break up and distribute evenly) with other ingredients.

Take extra time while mixing (1-2 minutes extra), slowly drizzling in the oil, and you shouldn't have a problem.

Salmonella contamination from raw eggs is a risk worthy of note. We have taken this risk for 20 years without one problem as we buy our eggs from a local farm. If you're concerned about salmonella, purchase pasteurized eggs or pasteurize them yourself at home by giving the eggs a 5 minute bath in 131°F water (the white may slightly cook, but the yolk inside remains viable).

On average, correctly made and stored mayonnaise remains fresh for 7-10 days. Ours always gets eaten before a week passes. Note the expiry date of eggs on your mayonnaise container – the egg portion of your mayonnaise is your only cause for concern.

KetoHybrid Mayo

Scale this recipe up or down based on your needs.

Yield: 24 servings or approximately 1 1/2 cups
Serving Size: 1 tablespoon
Nutrition: 0.1 net carb
Prep Time: 3 to 5 minutes

2 egg yolks
1 tsp Dijon-style mustard
2 tsp lemon juice
1 tbsp white wine vinegar
1/2 tsp salt
pinch of cayenne pepper
1 cup olive oil

Amount Per Serving	
Calories	84.35
Calories From Fat (98%)	82.96

Total Fat 9.38g	
Saturated Fat 1.38g	
Cholesterol 15.01mg	
Sodium 51.91mg	
Potassium 2.94mg	
Total Carbohydrates 0.13g	
Fiber 0.01g	
Sugar 0.02g	
Protein 0.23g	

98%   1%

KetoHybrid
2014

1. Briefly blend all ingredients except oil in a food processor or blender on low setting (30 seconds).
2. Slowly drizzle in the oil with the mixer still running (if your blender allows) on low (2-3 minutes).
3. Once all ingredients have been added and the mayonnaise has firmed up, you can add a teaspoon of distilled water (boiled and cooled water) to thin it if you like.
4. Refrigerate.

Jean's* Coconut Oil Mayonnaise

There are hundreds of reasons why you should consider choosing virgin coconut oil over olive oil, but not everyone likes the taste. This recipe makes adding more coconut oil into your diet effortless.

Note: Due to the lack of vinegar in this recipe, the risk of salmonella is higher. Use pasteurized eggs only or consume this mayonnaise within a few days of creation. See previous page for details on salmonella and pasteurization.

Yield: 16 servings

Serving Size: 1 tablespoon

Net Carbs per Serving: 0.1 grams

Prep Time: 5-8 minutes

2 egg yolks

1/2 tbsp lemon juice

1/4 tsp dried mustard

pinch of salt

1/3 cup olive oil

1/3 cup coconut oil (slightly warmed to a semi-liquid state)

Amount Per Serving	
Calories	85.91
Calories From Fat (98%)	83.95

Total Fat 9.6g	
Saturated Fat 4.74g	
Cholesterol 22.51mg	98%
Sodium 5mg	
Potassium 3.37mg	
Total Carbohydrates 0.14g	
Fiber 0.01g	
Sugar 0.03g	KetoHybrid
Protein 0.35g	2014

1. Eggs need to be at room temperature to emulsify with coconut oil. One hour on the counter is usually sufficient.
2. Melt coconut oil to a liquid state to prevent clumping in your finished mayonnaise. Coconut oil turns to solid at 76°F.
3. Briefly blend all ingredients except oils in a food processor or blender on low setting (1 minutes).
4. Slowly drizzle in the oils with the mixer still running (if your blender allows) on low (2-3 minutes).
5. If the mayonnaise seems too thick, add a teaspoon of distilled water (boiled and cooled tap water if you don't have distilled water on hand). Refrigerate.

*Jean Armstrong wrote the book on coconut oil. She's been using it in her kitchen for over 20 years and has extensively researched the health benefits of using the oil as food, medicine and personal care products. Check out "Coconut Oil Miracle or Myth?[17]" (2014) for more recipes and information.

---

17 https://www.amazon.com/dp/B00IYCTC0A

Salad Dressings

Blue Cheese (aka Roquefort) Dip or Dressing

Great with chicken wings or as a salad dressing.

Yield: 7 servings

Serving size: 1 ounce

Net Carbs per Serving: 0.2 grams

Prep Time: 5 minutes

2 ounces blue cheese, room temperature, divided

1/2 cup sour cream

2 tbsp white wine vinegar

1/2 tsp salt

1/2 tsp celery seed

1/4 teaspoon tarragon

pinch garlic powder

pinch onion powder

pinch paprika

Amount Per Serving	
Calories	5.88
Calories From Fat (60%)	3.51

Total Fat 0.4g	
Saturated Fat 0.12g	
Cholesterol 12.87mg	
Sodium 24.7mg	
Potassium 9.16mg	
Total Carbohydrates 0.34g	
Fiber 0.1g	
Sugar 0.03g	
Protein 0.31g	

60%

20%

21%

KetoHybrid
2014

1. Reserving one ounce of the blue cheese, blend all other ingredients until smooth.
2. Crumble and fold in the remaining cheese.
3. Serve immediately or refrigerate up to the shelf life of your sour cream.

French Dressing

French salad dressing is traditionally a little sweet. For that reason I've added a small amount of sugar substitute. I am not a fan of French Dressing and can only recommend this version based on friends' input. If you think this version is lacking, or have suggestions to make it better, please email me at veronica@ketohybrid.com.

This recipe uses raw egg, please read the information on using raw eggs in the mayonnaise section (above).

Yield: 15 ounces
Serving Size: 1 ounce
Net Carbs per Serving: 0.5 grams
Prep Time: 5 minutes
Time to Table: 1 hour

Amount Per Serving	
Calories	132.37
Calories From Fat (95%)	126.38

Total Fat 14.31g	
Saturated Fat 4g	
Cholesterol 31.73mg	95%
Sodium 233.73mg	
Potassium 22.59mg	
Total Carbohydrates 0.62g	
Fiber 0.08g	
Sugar 0.06g	KetoHybrid
Protein 0.89g	2014

2 tsp Dijon-style mustard
1 1/2 tsp lemon juice
1 tsp garlic powder
1/2 tsp tarragon, dried
1/4 tsp white pepper
1/4 tsp onion powder
1/4 tsp paprika
1 tsp salt
1/4 tsp sugar substitute (or omit)
1/2 cup olive oil
1/2 cup heavy cream
1 raw egg

1. Combine all ingredients except egg and oil in a blender and process until smooth. Alternating – add in small amounts of egg yolk followed by small amounts of oil until fully blended.
2. Allow to rest in the refrigerator for one hour.
3. Serve immediately or use within a few days.

Green Goddess Dressing

Before Caesar salad dressing became so popular, the world adored the Green Goddess. If you've never tried it, this is the perfect opportunity to whip up a batch and impress your friends with a delicious retro dressing.

Yield: 7 ounces

Serving size: 1 ounce

Net Carbs per Serving: 0.5

Prep Time: 5 minutes

Time to Table: 30 minutes

1/2 cup homemade mayonnaise (nutrition calculated using coconut oil mayo above)

1 anchovy fillet (or 1⁄2 tsp anchovy paste)

1⁄4 tsp garlic powder

1 tbsp green onion, finely chopped

1 tbsp parsley, fresh and chopped

3 tbsp sour cream

1/4 tsp salt

1/8 tsp black pepper

Amount Per Serving	
Calories	110.51
Calories From Fat (96%)	105.59

Total Fat 12.07g	
Saturated Fat 6.04g	
Cholesterol 28.89mg	95%
Sodium 111.02mg	
Potassium 22.1mg	
Total Carbohydrates 0.56g	
Fiber 0.07g	
Sugar 0.26g	KetoHybrid
Protein 0.71g	2014

1. Combine all ingredients by hand. Let rest in the refrigerator for 30 minutes to blend flavors.
2. Use within 5-7 days (dependent upon expiry date of ingredients used).

Italian Salad Dressing

If you have fresh herbs, substitute them in equal quantities. This recipe also makes a delicious one-hour marinade for chicken or pork. Recipe scales up well.

Yield: 8 servings

Serving size: 1 ounce

Net Carbs per Serving: 1.1 grams

Prep Time: 5 minutes

Time to Table: 35 minutes

1⁄3 cup wine vinegar

2⁄3 cup olive oil

1⁄2 tsp salt

1 tsp garlic, minced

1 tsp oregano, dried

1 tsp rosemary, dried and rubbed or finely chopped

1 tsp basil, dried

pinch hot pepper flakes

1/4 tsp black pepper

1 ounce lemon juice

Amount Per Serving	
Calories	163.52
Calories From Fat (98%)	159.62
Total Fat 18.06g	
Saturated Fat 2.51g	
Cholesterol 0mg	
Sodium 146.17mg	
Potassium 24.8mg	
Total Carbohydrates 1.32g	
Fiber 0.24g	
Sugar 0.11g	
Protein 0.11g	

98%   0%

KetoHybrid
2014

1. Blend all spices in white wine vinegar and allow to stand for 30 minutes or more.
2. Mix in olive oil and lemon juice.
3. Shake before serving. Refrigerate up to 1 month.

KetoHybrid Caesar Salad (Dressing or Dip)

You could eat salad for breakfast, lunch, and dinner and still gain weight if you're dousing it in commercially prepared dressings. Nearly all are mass produced by manufacturers of questionable practices and come loaded with chemicals, sugar, and GMO oils. I must be careful not to bash all factory foods here – we still need the Worcestershire Sauce to make this dressing great!

Caesar Salad was once a specialty – long before it became the common staple it is today. In 5 star restaurants, a salad chef would arrive at your table to create his masterpiece. He'd begin by crushing garlic into a wooden bowl, and follow up with salt-cured anchovies, fresh yolks, the finest oil and freshly grated black pepper. Hand-torn lettuce leaves, croutons and more cheese finished the creation.

Since you don't have time for that level of pomp, we're including our favorite and fastest Caesar recipe below. We're using mayonnaise instead of the traditional raw egg (made with your own homemade mayo or a store variety) to keep it easy.

The recipe works wonderfully for a dinner salad; include lettuce, cheese and chopped bacon and the macros balance wonderfully. Top your salad with 4 ounces of grilled chicken if you need to increase protein intake for the day (30 grams protein per 4 ounces grilled chicken).

You can make this by hand (with a whisk) or by machine (food processor or hand blender). As with most dressings, add oil slowly while mixing to ensure even distribution – blending to a creamy consistency.

Yield: 9 ounces (6 side salads or 3 entree salads)
Serving Size: 1 1/2 ounces per side salad, 3 ounces per entree salad
Net Carbs per Serving: 2.2 grams per 1.5 ounces
Prep Time: 5 minutes

1/2 cup plus 2 tsp olive oil
3 tbsp mayonnaise (nutrition

Amount Per Serving	
Calories	229.31
Calories From Fat (90%)	206.52
Total Fat 23.38g	
Saturated Fat 3.8g	
Cholesterol 6.43mg	
Sodium 201.17mg	
Potassium 43.85mg	
Total Carbohydrates 3.63g	
Fiber 0.14g	
Sugar 0.83g	
Protein 2.26g	

90%

6%
4%

KetoHybrid
2014

calculated using grocery store mayonnaise)

1 tbsp dijon mustard

1 1/2 tbsp garlic, minced

1/4 cup Parmesan cheese, grated

1 1/2 tbsp anchovy paste

2 tbsp lemon juice

2 tsp Worcestershire sauce

1. Begin by mixing all ingredients together, except for the olive oil.
2. Slowly drizzle the oil while continuing to mix slowly. Five to seven minutes by hand, three to four minutes in a food processor or with a hand blender on low.

KetoHybrid Ranch (Dressing or Dip)

Yield: 1 cup

Serving Size: 1 ounce

Net Carbs per Serving: 3.1 grams

Prep Time: 5 minutes

1 cup mayonnaise

1/2 cup sour cream

1/2 cup cream cheese

3/4 tsp salt

1/2 tsp black pepper

1 tbsp onion powder

1 tsp garlic powder

1 tbsp dried parsley

1/4 tsp celery salt

1/2 tsp dried dill

1/2 tsp dried mustard powder

Amount Per Serving	
Calories	77.59
Calories From Fat (78%)	60.65
Total Fat 6.89g	
Saturated Fat 2.87g	
Cholesterol 14.86mg	
Sodium 230.06mg	
Potassium 45.56mg	
Total Carbohydrates 3.5g	
Fiber 0.24g	
Sugar 1.11g	
Protein 0.94g	

78%
17%
5%

KetoHybrid 2014

1. Blend all ingredients together for a thick Ranch dip.
2. If using for a salad dressing, add 1/2 ounce of water or buttermilk for every ounce of dip.

Nutritional information given for dip – adjust as necessary for salad dressing.

Alfredo Sauce

The easy version of a creamy white cheese sauce traditionally served on fettucini, and is perfect for zucchini noodles, or chicken and fish.

A scoop of Alfredo adds ample fat and flavor to many meals. Make it yours by adding your favorites to create an entire meal. We pour it on 8 cups of zucchini noodles and 8 ounces of cooked chicken for four (3 cup, 400 calories, 7.7 net carb, 65F-25P-9C) dinner meals.

Yield: 4 servings
Serving Size: 1/4 cup
Net Carbs per Serving: 2.5 grams
Prep Time: 5 minutes
Cook Time: 3-7 minutes

1 tbsp butter
2 tsp garlic, minced
1 cup heavy cream
1/3 cup Parmesan cheese, grated
1/8 tsp nutmeg
1/4 tsp salt
1/4 tsp black pepper

Amount Per Serving	
Calories	269.42
Calories From Fat (89%)	240.19
Total Fat 27.31g	
Saturated Fat 16.99g	
Cholesterol 96.48mg	
Sodium 296.03mg	
Potassium 63.52mg	
Total Carbohydrates 2.58g	
Fiber 0.08g	
Sugar 0.18g	
Protein 4.56g	

89%

KetoHybrid
2014

1. In a large skillet over medium heat, lightly saute garlic in butter (1 minute), then add the cream and gently heat through.
2. Stir Parmesan cheese in slowly, then spices, while continuing to stir.
3. The sauce will begin to thicken quickly (turn to medium-low if necessary to ensure the sauce doesn't stick, boil, or burn). Continue stirring until the sauce is consistent in texture, slightly thinner than mayonnaise.
4. Can be stored in the refrigerator up to 1 week and re-heated gently in the microwave.

Blender Hollandaise Sauce

Few people make perfect Hollandaise Sauce on their first attempt. Once you've got the hang of it, you'll turn often to Hollandiase as it is a delicious way to increase fats for meals containing eggs, fish, chicken, or vegetables.

The most common mistake is in the butter temperature. Butter cools quickly so if you've started blending the eggs with the butter and the sauce isn't thickening up, you'll have to turn up the heat. To do so, transfer the sauce to a small pan and cook over very low heat for a few minutes while whisking. Great chefs make Hollandaise in a double boiler but for small batches and with careful attention, you won't need to. You can also try this in the microwave but it is a practice of finesse – heat too quickly and too hot and the sauce will separate, cooking the eggs in the process. However, if you have a helper willing to stand at the microwave door for 2 minutes, removing and whisking every 8 seconds, the microwave is an option.

Even if the sauce isn't perfect in your first few attempts, eat it anyway. While it may not present well, it will still taste great! I promise you that your second batch (or perhaps third) will be perfect.

Store extra sauce in the refrigerator, covered, for 3-5 days. Reheat gently on the stove or in the microwave.

Yield: Almost 1 cup

Serving Size: 3 tablespoons

Net Carbs per Serving: 0.7 grams

Prep Time: 5 minutes

Cook Time: 10 minutes

3 egg yolks

4 ounces unsalted butter, melted

1/4 tsp salt (omit if using salted butter)

1 tbsp lemon juice

1 tbsp water

pinch of cayenne

Amount Per Serving	
Calories	244.47
Calories From Fat (95%)	232.3
Total Fat 26.33g	
Saturated Fat 15.77g	
Cholesterol 196.09mg	
Sodium 154.6mg	
Potassium 24.94mg	
Total Carbohydrates 0.74g	
Fiber 0.02g	
Sugar 0.19g	
Protein 2.23g	

95%

KetoHybrid
2014

1. In a small bowl or pan, melt the butter, then add lemon juice and water.
2. In a small blender, mix egg yolks thoroughly with salt, pepper, and cayenne – about 30 seconds. Immediately begin drizzling the warmed butter into the blender, ensuring that the blender is still running.
3. As the two (butter and eggs) emulsify the sauce begins to thicken – about 1-2 minutes.
4. Serve immediately or refrigerate up to 5 days.

Low Carb Tartar Sauce

You'll never want to eat commercially-prepared tartar sauce again.

Yield: 10 servings

Serving Size: 1 tablespoon

Net Carbs per Serving: 0.1 grams

Prep Time: 5 minutes

1/2 cup of homemade coconut oil mayonnaise

2 tsp capers, chopped and drained

1 tsp chives, fresh and minced (or dried if not in season)

1 tsp lemon juice

1 tbsp dill pickles, finely chopped

Amount Per Serving	
Calories	69.3
Calories From Fat (97%)	67.41

Total Fat 7.71g	
Saturated Fat 3.81g	
Cholesterol 18.01mg	
Sodium 29.48mg	
Potassium 4.63mg	
Total Carbohydrates 0.2g	
Fiber 0.04g	
Sugar 0.05g	
Protein 0.3g	

97%

KetoHybrid
2014

1. Combine all ingredients.
2. Refrigerate up to the shelf date of your mayonnaise.

KetoHybrid Tzatziki

Yet another favorite from the island of Greece! This creamy dip works overtime on meats as well as vegetables. Perfect to pour over pork or chicken shish-kebobs, or enjoy as a cracker or vegetable dip.

Tzatziki is traditionally made with Greek yogurt. Commercially prepared Greek yogurt averages 1 carb (0 fiber) per tablespoon. If you're a person who can stop at one tablespoon, you won't need this recipe, but if you're like us, you'd be happier with 3 or 4 tablespoons for the same amount of net carbs.

Enter the KetoHybid Tzatziki! Our home version that quarters those carbs, has the same tangy bite and is wonderfully creamy. You may never glance at a tub of Greek yogurt again...

Yield: 10 servings
Serving Size: 2 ounces (4 tablespoons)
Net Carbohydrates: 1.4 grams
Prep Time: 10 minutes
Time to Table: 30 minutes

1 cup sour cream
1/2 cup ricotta cheese
1 cup cucumber, peeled, seeded and coarsely chopped
1 1/2 tsp garlic, minced
1/2 tsp salt
2 tsp dill, fresh, chopped

Amount Per Serving	
Calories	68.03
Calories From Fat (79%)	54.05

Total Fat 6.16g	
Saturated Fat 3.67g	
Cholesterol 18.23mg	
Sodium 145.37mg	
Potassium 65.41mg	
Total Carbohydrates 1.47g	
Fiber 0.1g	
Sugar 1.03g	
Protein 1.97g	

79%
8%
12%

KetoHybrid
2014

1. Place cucumber pieces in a colander. Liberally shake salt over the cucumber and allow to drain for 20 minutes.
2. Add all other ingredients to blender and process until smooth (2-3 minutes).
3. Shake remaining salt off cucumbers and add to the blender.
4. Use the pulse or chop setting until no large chunks of cucumber can be found.
5. Store refrigerated in a glass container up to 1 week.

Crème Fraîche

If you've never had crème fraîche, allow me to introduce it to you. While it can not and should not replace other foods, it adds a new taste to your 'safe' foods.

Crème Fraîche is a dairy food with a texture and taste best imagined between yogurt and sour cream; without the tangy taste. It is creamier and has a higher fat content than sour cream or yogurt. When made at home, it is 50% lower in carbs than either dairy product. Crème Fraîche can be purchased in most grocery stores but is certainly higher in carbohydrates than the recipe below.

Should you make it, and like it, you can eat it in a variety of ways. With a few berries (yogurt), in dips or dressings (think sour cream), in potato, egg, or tuna salad (think mayonnaise), or in any creamy sauces or soups (it won't curdle like cream or sour cream when heated).

Many people leave their Crème Fraîche out on the counter, but we refrigerate ours. Crème fraîche stays fresh for several weeks.

While I haven't used it in any recipes within the book – make Crème Fraîche just once at home and I think you'll find many uses for it. Here's an example: Increase the creaminess of our Faux Mac and Cheese by adding 3 ounces of Crème Fraîche to the recipe; net carbs will only be increased by 1.5g for the entire recipe.

The following recipe makes 1 cup, enough for you to try it and have a starter to work from. We've also laid out the nutritional data for a 3 ounce serving so you can quickly adapt your favorite recipes.

Serving Size: 3 ounces
Net Carbs per Serving: 1.5 grams
Prep Time: 5 minutes
Passive Time: 2-12 hours

1 cup heavy cream
1 tsp cultured buttermilk

1. In a small saucepan over low heat, gently warm heavy cream until slightly warm to your touch.
2. Add buttermilk and stir to combine.

3. Pour into a glass or ceramic jar with a tight lid and leave out on the counter until it thickens (a minimum of 12 hours and up to 2 days).
4. When the starter has reached the desired consistency, stir and refrigerate.
5. Similar to sourdough starters (if you've baked bread in the past), you can continue making Crème Fraîche by using a portion of your initial batch. Add two tablespoons of a previous Crème Fraîche to two cups of fresh cream and leave out on the counter until the right consistency.

Creamy Comparisons: 100 ml = 3 oz = 6 tablespoons

Crème Fraîche - 165 calories, 16.5 g fat, 1.5 g carbs, 1.5 g protein
Whipping cream (nothing added) - 284 cal, 30 g fat, 3 g carbs, 1 g protein
Yogurt (whole milk) - 42 cal, 3 g fat, 3 g carbs, 3 g protein
Sour Cream - 162 cal, 18 g fat, 3 g carbs, 3 g protein

HOW TO GET
A 2 WEEK MEAL PLAN... FREE
OR 20 MORE RECIPES...

Send a photo of yourself holding this book and we'll send along your choice of either book for free!

Get The Details - www.KetoHybrid.com/freebook

Rubs & Marinades

Just like mayonnaise and other condiments, spice blends and marinades are known for having questionable ingredients within the packaging. Studies have found both sugar and sawdust mixed into spice blends to bulk up the jar and make you feel you're getting value for the extra volume. A blend can be inexpensively created in your own kitchen, with better quality control.

Here are a few of our favorites to get you started.

Steak Rub

Perfect for barbequed steaks or chops. This rub only enhances - never masks – the flavor of your main dish.

Yield: 20+ servings
Net Carbs per Serving: 0.9 grams*
Prep Time: 5 minutes

3 tbsp paprika
1 tbsp garlic powder
1 tbsp onion powder
1 tbsp crushed coriander
1 tsp crushed red pepper
2 tbsp salt
1 tbsp black pepper

1. Mix together.
2. Store in a glass jar at room temperature.
3. Rub onto meat and allow to soak in 1-6 hours or use immediately before grilling.

*Theoretically this rub adds 1 net carb per serving, but it is my belief that these spices cook off upon grilling – providing lots of extra flavor without adding extra carbs.

Blackening Spice

Rub this spice into thin fillets of chicken, pork or fish before pan frying. The spice darkens as the protein cooks – adding a delicious smokey flavor to your dinner.

Yield: 20+ servings
Prep Time: 5 minutes
Net Carbs per Serving: 0.9 grams

5 tbsp paprika
1 tbsp dried thyme
1 tbsp black pepper
1 tbsp garlic powder
1/2 tsp cayenne pepper
5 tbsp salt
1/2 tsp ground white pepper

Shish KeBab Marinade

A simple marinade for pork or chicken shish-kebabs.

Yield: Enough for 3 pounds of meat before skewering
Serving Size: 1/6 recipe
Net Carbs per Serving: 1.3 grams*
Prep Time: 10 minutes
Time to Table: 3 to 6 hours

2 tbsp olive oil
2 tbsp garlic, minced
2 tbsp oregano, fresh, chopped
2 tbsp red onion, finely chopped
1 1/2 tsp salt
1 tsp black pepper

1. Mix all ingredients together and marinate kebab cubes, refrigerated, in a covered glass container for 3-6 hours before grilling.

*Adding 1.3 grams of net carbs per serving may seem high, but most of that count is derived from the onions and garlic; two items that will be cooked off or left behind during the grilling process.

Ginger Marinade

Another great marinade for chicken, pork or fish.

Yield: Enough for 2 1/2 to 3 pounds of meat
Serving Size: 1/5 to 1/6 recipe
Net Carbs per Entire Recipe: 2.9 grams if cooked into the meal
Prep Time: 10 minutes
Time to Table: 2 to 12 hours

1/4 cup extra virgin olive oil
3 tbsp red wine vinegar
1 1/2 tbsp fresh ginger, peeled and grated
1 tbsp rosemary
1/2 tsp garlic, minced
1/4 tsp crushed red pepper flakes
1/2 tsp salt
1/4 tsp black pepper

1. Mix all ingredients together and set aside 1/3 cup of finished marinade.
2. Pour remaining 2/3 over your chicken, fish or pork and refrigerate from 2-12 hours before cooking.
3. Cook the meat in your marinade if you like, but do not reserve uncooked, used marinade for a later date.

CHAPTER 23

Desserts

Kicking a dessert habit to the curb is difficult, so if you're suffering we do hope this chapter takes away some of the sting.

Like the informational chapter on sugar and substitutes, Veronica has allowed me to write this chapter exclusively. In truth, I wanted to omit desserts from this book; it would be best if you never thought of them again.

If I could live on sugar and desserts alone, I'd be the happiest human on planet earth. However, desserts are best left to very special occasions and in moderation. Once or twice a year a small piece of birthday cake is appropriate; some sherbert on the hottest afternoon of summer; a true Italian cannoli enjoyed on a trip to Tuscany – you get my point right?

Unfortunately I can quickly turn one scoop of ice cream on the occasional Sunday afternoon into three scoops every summer evening. The same is true for birthday cake. If I make a cake of healthy ingredients I seem to think I have free license to eat the whole cake; which I've done in the past. Yes, I have a problem.

"There's a cake made of healthy ingredients?" There are many that claim to be, and we've made more than a few trying to a pleasant balance of nutrition and taste. You'll see a few below, but first we need to talk about our definition of healthy.

KetoHybrid defines healthy foods as being all natural with no chemical processes or additives. To keep it low carb, our selection becomes a few berries or slices of melon. In moments of weakness when we first started this diet we would make desserts sweetened with raw sugar or honey. This was counter-productive for the fat burning switch of KetoHybrid, but it was marginally better than blowing carb counts with pre-made, pre-packaged, desserts.

You've no doubt read the earlier chapter on sugar substitutes. Whether they cause cancer, elevate blood sugar, wreak havoc on your metabolism, create new addictions, increase the risk of heart disease, are made from natural sources, or not – they're better left alone.

The good news is that within a few weeks your taste buds and cravings will have changed. Today, Veronica finds the taste of sweetness to be revolting. I haven't gotten that far but I am noticing that even carrots taste unpleasantly sweet lately.

All posturing aside though, we both remember what the cravings were like in the beginning. For that reason we are including some of our best desserts – to be eaten in moderation – that incorporate both low carb and high fat. We leave the decision to you as to how you sweeten each recipe, adjusting by taste and altering the carb macro if necessary. If you need help, just drop me an email at laura@ketohybrid.com.

Flavor Drops & Extracts

Many diet forums suggest adding flavor drops to foods since they contain less (or none) carbs per serving than their natural counterpart. You'll find these references as a way to supplement whey protein powder in smoothies, or in baking. On the surface, this is a good idea, but before you head out to purchase a bottle in every delicious flavor, I have some valuable information for you.

Throughout our research we've become extremely picky about these drops, even when labeled sugar free or low carb. Many contain propylene glycol - a chemical compound passed by North American governments as GRAS (generally regarded as safe). Propylene glycol isn't just in flavor extracts, you'll also find it in prepared foodstuffs – from ice cream to baked goods to bottled beer – often in small enough amounts that manufacturers aren't required to list it on the label as anything other than "flavor extracts".

While propylene glycol may be considered safe and you may be using just a few drops on occasion, I would steer clear of it. Propylene glycol is the 'medicine' large feedlots give to cattle to prevent ketosis – it actually prevents animals from burning fat for fuel (the opposite of what you're working so hard to accomplish with your KetoHybrid diet).

Everything we eat comes with an ounce of risk – especially so when it isn't a whole and natural food that has been raised or grown organically. My aim is to help you make educated choices so you can balance the risks of cost, carbs, health, flavor and satiety. To that end, beginning on June 15, 2014, we will begin list creation of companies and products that we consider both safe and suitable for the KetoHybrid diet.

Any Berry Syrup

Yield: 1 cup

Serving Size: 1/4 cup

Net Carbs per Serving: Blackberry: 1.56 g, Blueberry: 4.4 g, Raspberry: 1.69 g, Strawberry: 2.17

Prep Time: 5 minutes

Cook Time: 5-10 minutes

1 cup fresh berries

1/2 cup water

1/2 teaspoon xanthan powder or guar gum

Stevia or sugar substitute to taste (only if required)

Amount Per Serving	
Calories	16.45
Calories From Fat (6%)	0.96
Total Fat 0.12g	
Saturated Fat 0.01g	
Cholesterol 0mg	
Sodium 37.39mg	
Potassium 63.05mg	
Total Carbohydrates 3.92g	
Fiber 1.75g	
Sugar 1.86g	
Protein 0.26g	

KetoHybrid 2014

1. Puree fresh berries and water in a blender.
2. Transfer berries from the blender to a small pan over low heat. Stir in guar gum or xanthan powder and continue to stir until sauce thickens.
3. You may need to increase heat slightly, add an extra measure of guar or xanthan (to make it thicker), or a bit of water (if thickened too much).
4. Once you reach the perfect consistency, keep the heat low and add a few drops of stevia or sweetener if required.
5. Refrigerate up to 10 days.

Strawberry version shown in nutrition data above.

Quick Berry Jam

If you're already reading nutrition labels at the grocery store, you've figured out that a low carb high fat diet doesn't include jam. While that may be true for most 'low-carbers', I've got some great news for you!

Jam – if made at home using the recipe below – is safe to add to your diet.

Before you go skipping off to the kitchen, a basket of freshly picked strawberries on your arm, read this section on why you should never eat any other homemade or commercially prepared jam. Even jam labeled sugar free should be off limits.

Jam is traditionally made with plenty of sugar and a little pectin. Here's the formula, loosely calculated from one of the top home canning websites.

13 parts berries - 1 part pectin - 18 parts sugar

It is easy to see that every tablespoon of jam has more sugar than berry.

Sugar – 48 calories and 12.6 carbohydrates per tablespoon – absolutely ruins jams for us.

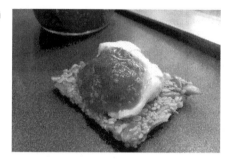

Pectin – a natural product that shortens the cook time and increases shelf life – also has a negative effect, even in such small quantities.

Pectin per tablespoon: 46 calories, 12.8 carbohydrates, 1.2 fiber, 11.6 net carbs.

I'm skipping ahead but you can trust I've done the math. Sugar-hate aside, the small bit of pectin in a recipe adds 10 calories and 1 net carb to every tablespoon of jam – more than doubling the caloric count, and nearly doubling net carbs.

And while that extra gram of carbohydrate may not seem a big deal on paper, if I were to ask you whether you'd rather have 1 or 2 tablespoons of strawberry jam with your crepes, which would you choose?

The good news is that you don't have to give up having a little jam every now and then. You just need to make it yourself in a nontraditional manner.

For this, you'll need chia seeds (aka Salvia hispanica), found at health food stores or online. One tablespoon of chia has 69 calories, 2 grams of protein, 4.5 grams fat, 6 grams carbohydrates, 5.5 grams of fiber, and 0.5 net carbs. By using it you're adding fat, you're adding protein, and even though you're adding a few extra calories, what you're saving is 11+ net carbs when compared to pectin. For the low carb dieter, these little seeds are a dream come true.

When chia seeds meet with a liquid, they soften to a gel-like consistency and bind nearby ingredients to each other. Like you might need in gravy. Or meatballs. But best of all, in an all-natural, sugar free jam.

All Natural Sugar Free Jam

Serving Size: 1 tablespoon
Net Carbs per serving: 1.2 g
Yield: 8 servings

1 cup strawberries, chopped
1 tbsp water
1 tbsp chia seeds

Amount Per Serving	
Calories	14.76
Calories From Fat (34%)	5.03
Total Fat 0.6g	
Saturated Fat 0.06g	
Cholesterol 0mg	
Sodium 0.53mg	
Potassium 31.91mg	
Total Carbohydrates 2.24g	
Fiber 1.05g	
Sugar 0.93g	
Protein 0.4g	

KetoHybrid 2014

1. Add clean, chopped strawberries with 1 tablespoon of water to a small pan over medium-high heat and bring to a slow boil. (Omit water if using frozen strawberries.)
2. Remove from heat as soon as berries soften (4-5 minutes) and mash to desired consistency.
3. Add chia seeds and sweetener (if you really think you must use sweetener) and mix well.
4. Let rest 15 minutes, stir again and transfer to a glass jar.
5. Refrigerate and use within 2 weeks.

Comparison fruits and berries (1 cup measure) that make delicious fresh jam:
Apricot: 79 calories, 18.4 g carbohydrate, 5.1 g net carbs
Peach: 66 calories, 16.2 g carbohydrate, 13.7 net carbs
Blackberry: 62 calories, 13.8 g carbohydrate, 6.2 net carbs
Blueberry: 84 calories, 21.5 g carbohydrate, 17.9 net carbs
Strawberry: 53 calories, 12.8 g carbohydrate, 9.5 net carbs
Raspberry: 64 calories, 14.7 g carbohydrate, 6.7 net carbs
Rhubarb: 26 calories, 5.5 g carbohydrate, 3.3 net carbs

A to Z Cinnamon Loaf

This recipe makes a moist loaf that works best as a vehicle for cream cheese or all natural jam.

Yield: Twelve slices, 2 mini loaves
Serving Size: 1 slice or 1/6 of a loaf
Net Carbs per Serving: 3.8 g per slice
Prep time: 10 minutes
Cook time: 35 minutes

1 1/2 cups almond flour

1 1/2 tsp baking soda

1/2 tsp salt

2 tsp cinnamon

1 1/4 cup zucchini, peel and grated (about two 6" young zucchini)

3 eggs

1 tsp vanilla extract

2 tbsp sugar substitute

1/3 cup mashed banana* (about one 6"-7" banana)

1 tbsp coconut oil, melted (or butter)

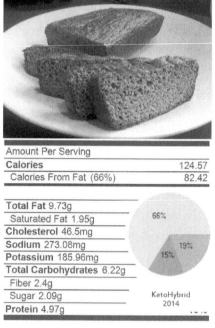

Amount Per Serving	
Calories	124.57
Calories From Fat (66%)	82.42
Total Fat 9.73g	
Saturated Fat 1.95g	
Cholesterol 46.5mg	
Sodium 273.08mg	
Potassium 185.96mg	
Total Carbohydrates 6.22g	
Fiber 2.4g	
Sugar 2.09g	
Protein 4.97g	

KetoHybrid 2014

1. Preheat oven to 350°F and lightly oil two non-stick, mini loaf pans – 7 x 3.5".
2. In a small bowl, combine dry ingredients.
3. Squeeze grated zucchini by hand or wring out in a clean kitchen towel to remove some of the water.
4. Process or blend all wet ingredients, except for zucchini, and mix for 2 minutes. Add zucchini to the food processor and mix, 2 minutes more.
5. Pour dry ingredients into the food processor and mix, 2 minutes more.
6. Divide batter into 2 equal portions (1 1/4 cup each) and pour into loaf pans.
7. Bake for 35 minutes, or until a toothpick comes out clean.
8. Cool 5 minutes before removing from pans. Cool loaves five minutes more on wire rack before slicing.

Substitute an equal amount of homemade applesauce or pumpkin puree but add a 1/4 tsp of banana flavoring to heighten flavor if you've found a healthy source.

Blueberry Dream Scones

These travel well. Make with any berry; the change in net carbs will be negligible. Raspberry version is the second set of nutritional information.

Calories and Net Carbs for A Blueberry Scone:

- Popular USA coffee shop chain: 460 calories and 65 g net carbs.
- KetoHybrid made with white sugar: 147.2 calories and 8.9 g net carbs (not shown)
- KetoHybrid made with zero-calorie sugar substitute: 122.8 calories and 3.9 g net carbs.

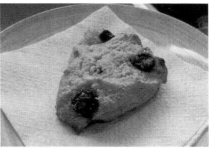

Yield: 6

Serving Size: 1 scone

Net Carbs per Serving: 3.9

Prep time: 5 minutes

Cook time: 15 minutes

2 eggs, beaten

1 cup almond flour

1/3 cup sugar substitute

1 1/2 tsp baking powder

1 1/2 tsp vanilla extract

1/2 cup fresh blueberries

Amount Per Serving	
Calories	148.16
Calories From Fat (65%)	96.42

Total Fat 11.41g	65%
Saturated Fat 1.26g	
Cholesterol 62mg	
Sodium 145.98mg	17%
Potassium 173.62mg	16%
Total Carbohydrates 6.61g	
Fiber 2.71g	
Sugar 2.17g	KetoHybrid
Protein 6.38g	2014

Amount Per Serving	
Calories	122.83
Calories From Fat (65%)	80.27

Total Fat 9.48g	65%
Saturated Fat 1.11g	
Cholesterol 62mg	
Sodium 145.89mg	16%
Potassium 151.37mg	17%
Total Carbohydrates 5.18g	
Fiber 2.6g	
Sugar 1.22g	KetoHybrid
Protein 5.58g	2014

1. Preheat oven to 375°F. Oil a non-stick baking sheet.
2. In a medium bowl, combine all ingredients, except blueberries, and mix well. If the dough appears too wet to shape, add a tablespoon more almond flour.
3. Gently fold in blueberries and split the batter into 6 equal portions. Shape each portion into traditional scone triangles, approximately 1" high, and place on baking sheet.
4. Bake until scones are lightly brown (about 15 minutes). Allow to cool on the pan for 5-10 minutes before serving.

KetoHybrid Cookies

A cookie dough that just plain works. On it's own it has a lovely buttery, nutty flavor. Add to it – adjusting macro-nutrients and net carbs – to make it your next favorite cookie.

We have made these with a few slivered almonds on top and find that they are both pretty and delicious. You might also add a few low-carb dark chocolate chips per cookie, or spice the entire batch with 1/2 tsp ginger, 1/4 tsp cloves and 1 tsp cinnamon for a yummy gingersnap cookie.

Yield: 24 1 1/2" cookies
Net Carbs per Serving: 0.6 grams
Serving Size: 4 cookies
Prep Time: 5 minutes
Bake Time: 15 minutes

2 cups almond flour
2 tbsp coconut flour
½ tsp xanthan gum
¼ tsp salt
1/4 tsp baking soda
6 tbsp butter, softened
1 large egg
½ tsp vanilla extract
½ cup sugar substitute

Amount Per Serving	
Calories	177.51
Calories From Fat (33%)	59.03
Total Fat 16.81g	
Saturated Fat 7.92g	
Cholesterol 61.53mg	
Sodium 183.08mg	
Potassium 15.48mg	
Total Carbohydrates 2.83g	
Fiber 2.37g	
Sugar 0.15g	
Protein 3.83g	

33%
17%
0%
50%

KetoHybrid
2014

1. Preheat oven to 350°F. Lightly oil a non-stick cookie sheet.
2. Blend all dry ingredients together.
3. Soften butter (in the microwave for 30 seconds if required) and blend with sugar substitute, egg, and vanilla extract. Add to the dry mixture.
4. Shape 24 slightly rounded teaspoonfuls into balls and lightly flatten to 1/4". Allow 1/4" spacing between cookies.
5. Bake 12-15 minutes or until cookies have turned a light golden color on edges.
6. Cool for 5 minutes on the sheet before removing.

Sugar-Free Whipped Cream

Yield: 2 cups (32 tablespoons)
Serving Size: 2 tablespoons
Net Carbs per Serving: 0.5
Prep Time: 4-6 minutes

1 cup cream, heavy or whipping
1/3 cup sugar substitute
1 tsp vanilla extract

1. Whip cold heavy cream with an electric mixer until frothy (3-4 minutes).
2. Add sugar substitute and vanilla extract. Whip on high until soft peaks form and cream has doubled in size (4-6 minutes).
3. Refrigerate excess topping in a sealed glass container for 7-10 days.

Amount Per Serving	
Calories	52.07
Calories From Fat (93%)	48.41

Total Fat 5.5g	
Saturated Fat 3.43g	
Cholesterol 20.38mg	93%
Sodium 5.68mg	
Potassium 11.54mg	
Total Carbohydrates 0.45g	
Fiber 0g	
Sugar 0.05g	KetoHybrid
Protein 0.31g	2014

KetoHybrid Mini Chocolate Cheesecake

Lovely and rich! Like a mug cake, only better. You can make these in a coffee mug, but they present better when cooked in little silicone baking cups.

Yield: 1 mini cake, 3 1/2" by 3 1/2"
Net Carbs per Serving: 4.2 g
Prep Time: 5 minutes
Cook Time: Less than 3 minutes

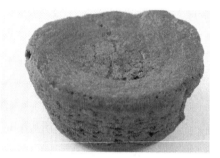

1 tsp butter
1 tbsp unsweetened cocoa powder
1/8 tsp baking powder
3 tsp sugar substitute
1 egg, beaten
1/2 tsp vanilla extract
1 tsp sour cream
2 oz softened cream cheese

1. In a small bowl, melt cream cheese (15 seconds in the microwave), add in vanilla and sour cream. Mix in the beaten egg.
2. Melt butter directly in a coffee mug (microwave for 10 seconds or less). Mix in dry ingredients.
3. Add cheese and egg mixture to the melted butter and cocoa mixture.
4. Microwave on high for 2 to 2 1/2 minutes. Allow to cool before eating.

Amount Per Serving	
Calories	322.43
Calories From Fat (82%)	263.59

Total Fat 29.88g	
Saturated Fat 13.83g	
Cholesterol 249.62mg	
Sodium 317.1mg	
Potassium 233.08mg	
Total Carbohydrates 6.02g	
Fiber 1.79g	
Sugar 2.18g	
Protein 10.75g	

82%

5%

14%

KetoHybrid
2014

Summer Lime Cake

This cake tastes the way that summer feels. When evening cravings strike, we will often just take a walk around the block. When it's raining and dismal we make one of these cakes and split it between us.

Yield: 1 cake, 4" x 4"
Serving Size: Entire recipe (but can easily satisfy two people)
Net Carbs per Serving: 3.1 grams
Prep Time: 3 minutes
Cook Time: Less than 2 minutes

1 tbsp butter, melted
2 eggs, beaten
2 tbsp sugar substitute
1 tbsp lime juice
1 tsp lime zest, grated
2 tbsp golden flax meal
2 tbsp almond flour
½ tsp baking powder

1. Melt butter directly in a ramekin or glass dish – about 10 seconds in microwave.
2. Stir in eggs, lime juice and zest.
3. Add remaining ingredients, mixing until smooth.
4. Microwave on high for 1 1/2 – 2 minutes or until set.

Amount Per Serving	
Calories	399.5
Calories From Fat (72%)	287.31

Total Fat 32.84g	
Saturated Fat 11.3g	72%
Cholesterol 402.53mg	
Sodium 394.99mg	10%
Potassium 358.18mg	19%
Total Carbohydrates 10.19g	
Fiber 7.11g	
Sugar 1.01g	KetoHybrid
Protein 18g	2014

Three Minute Muffin

Running out the door without breakfast again? Don't do it. Lunch is hours away and you've got a busy morning planned. For these days, try the three minute muffin – made with black raspberries but you can substitute any berry with minimal change in net carbs.

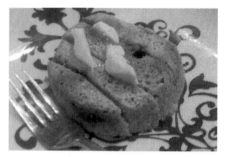

Yield: One 4" x 2" muffin
Net Carbs per Serving: 2.5 g
Prep Time: 1-2 minutes
Cook Time: Less than 2 minutes

1/4 cup golden flax seeds, ground
1/2 tsp baking powder
1 tsp low-carb sugar substitute
1/2 ounce raspberries (7-8 berries)
1 egg
1/4 tsp vanilla extract
1 tbsp coconut oil, warmed

1. Mix dry ingredients together in a ramekin or small glass bowl.
2. Beat in egg, warmed coconut oil and vanilla extract.
3. Gently fold in berries and microwave for approximately 2 minutes.

Amount Per Serving	
Calories	407.27
Calories From Fat (73%)	297.6

Total Fat 34.78g	
Saturated Fat 14.75g	73%
Cholesterol 186mg	
Sodium 326.66mg	13%
Potassium 407.46mg	13%
Total Carbohydrates 14.01g	
Fiber 11.5g	
Sugar 1.54g	KetoHybrid 2014
Protein 13.54g	

Made in the USA
Lexington, KY
27 April 2015